Patients With Cancer

UNDERSTANDING THE
PSYCHOLOGICAL PAIN

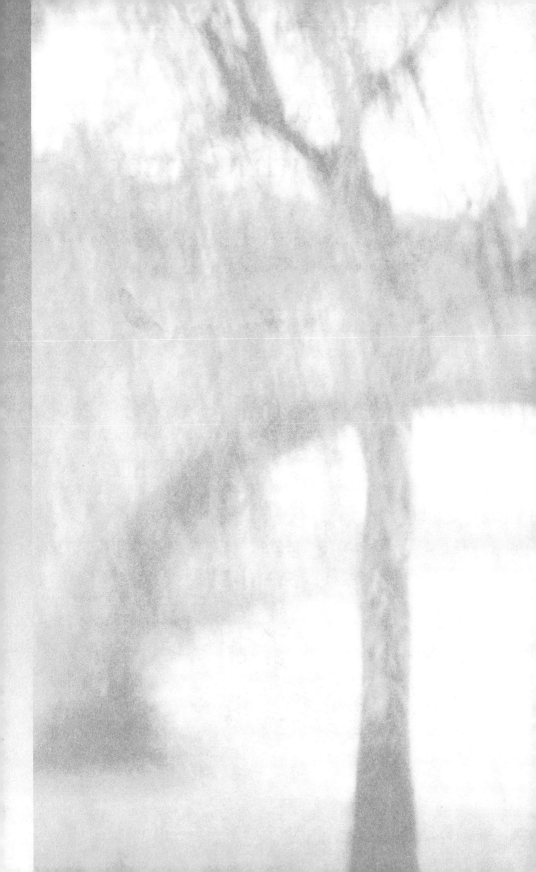

Patients
With Cancer

UNDERSTANDING THE
PSYCHOLOGICAL PAIN

Arlene D. Houldin, RN, PhD, CS
Associate Professor, Psychosocial Oncology Nursing
School of Nursing
University of Pennsylvania
Psychological Consultant, Cancer Center
Philadelphia, Pennsylvania

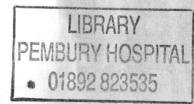
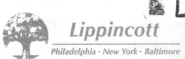
Lippincott
Philadelphia · New York · Baltimore

Sponsoring Editor: Jennifer Brogan
Editorial Assistant: Hilarie Surrena
Senior Project Editor: Sandra Cherrey Scheinin
Senior Production Manager: Helen Ewan

Production Coordinator: Patricia McCloskey
Art Director: Carolyn O'Brien
Indexer: Michael Ferreira
Manufacturing Manager: William Alberti

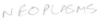

NEOPLASMS   PAIN PSYCHOLOGY
QZ 200 ?

9 8 7 6 5 4 3 2 1

Library of Congress Cataloging-in-Publication Data
Houldin, Arlene DeGangi.
    Patients with cancer : understanding the psychological pain / Arlene D. Houldin.
        p. ; cm.
    Includes bibliographical references and index.
    ISBN 0-7817-2020-6 (alk. paper)
        1. Cancer—Psychological aspects. 2. Cancer pain. I. Title.
        [DNLM: 1. Neoplasms—psychology. QZ 200 H838p 2000]
    RC262 .H686 2000
    616.99'4'9918—dc21   00-020041

Care has been taken to confirm the accuracy of the information presented and to describe generally accepted practices. However, the authors, editors, and publisher are not responsible for errors or omissions or for any consequences from application of the information in this book and make no warranty, express or implied, with respect to the contents of the publication.

The authors, editors and publisher have exerted every effort to ensure that drug selection and dosage set forth in this text are in accordance with current recommendations and practice at the time of publication. However, in view of ongoing research, changes in government regulations, and the constant flow of information relating to drug therapy and drug reactions, the reader is urged to check the package insert for each drug for any change in indications and dosage and for added warnings and precautions. This is particularly important when the recommended agent is a new or infrequently employed drug.

Some drugs and medical devices presented in this publication have Food and Drug Administration (FDA) clearance for limited use in restricted research settings. It is the responsibility of the health care provider to ascertain the FDA status of each drug or device planned for use in their clinical practice.

Artwork throughout this book was chosen from the University of Pennsylvania Cancer Center's "Confronting Cancer Through Art" exhibition, 1999.

*This book is dedicated to my patients,
both past and present, who have taught
me about courage, compassion, and the
preciousness of life.*

During the 10 years that I have worked in oncology, I have been privileged to witness and to share with my patients many occasions of upset and suffering, and equally as many of joy and laughter. As a result, I have been personally touched, taught, and transformed, gaining many insights that extend far beyond disease and pain. My motivation for writing this book was to share some of these insights with others in the hope of raising awareness of the personal, and too-often silent, concerns that individuals with cancer may face. Over the years, I have been struck by the similarities of these struggles among my patients. The first eight chapters of this book represent the themes that I have found repeatedly causing distress. Combining my personal experiential perspective as a clinician with the scholarly literature available on each topic, my goal was for this work to be well supported by the literature and well informed by the clinical wisdom gained from practice. As a result, the interventions taken from the theoretical review could be directly applicable to the realities of oncology practice today and useful for oncology clinicians to consider as a guide when supporting their patients through difficult times. The last chapter of the book is a concise compilation of select assessment and intervention techniques that are intended to be easily incorporated into practice settings.

CONTENTS

CHAPTER **1**

Where's the "Magic Bullet"? 1

Discussion of the Literature 2

Avoiding the Cookbook Recipes 2

Upset is Expected 3

Response Phases 3

Mind and Body Work 4

Psychoneuroimmunology Research Findings 5

Psychoneuroimmunology and Cancer 5

What Do the Findings Mean? 6

Clinical Implications 7

Answering Common Questions 7

The Perceptions of Our Patients 8

Normalize Distress 8

The Distress of Loved Ones 8

Contradicting Information 9

Clinical Strategies 9

Case Study 10

CHAPTER **2**

Denial 15

Discussion of the Literature 16

What is Denial? 16

Denial in Family Members 17

Denial in Staff 17

Denial: Process and Outcomes 18

Denial in Patients 18

Clinical Implications 19

Assessing Denial 19

When Denial Causes Problems 20

Perception of Denial 21

When Denial Protects Others 21

Promoting Denial 22

When Denial Interferes With Communication 22

Clinical Strategies 23

Case Study 23

CHAPTER **3**

Hope 27

Discussion of the Literature 28

Is Hope Always Adaptive? 28

Defining Hope 29

The Personal Experience of Hope 29

Hope in Patients With Cancer 30

Hope and Despair: Two Sides of the Coin 31

Clinical Implications 32

Assessment of Hope 33

Hope-Enhancing Strategies 33

Finding Hope Through the Presence of Others 34

Symptom Management Can Support Hope 34

Mindfulness Meditation 35

Supporting Personal Hopefulness 35

Other Unfulfilled Hopes 36

Clinicians' Contributions to Hopefulness 36

Communicating Bad News 37

Achieving a Delicate Balance 38

    Clinical Strategies 38

    Case Study 39

CHAPTER **4**

Uncertainty 43

Discussion of the Literature 44

    Illness-Related Uncertainty 44

    Personal Perception of Uncertainty 45

    Danger Versus Opportunity 45

    Coping Strategies 46

    An Uncertain World 47

    Patterns of Uncertainty 47

    An Uncertain Body 48

    Uncertainty and Social Support 49

    Complexity of Uncertainty 49

Clinical Implications 50

    Assessment of Uncertainty 50

    Individualized Plan of Support 51

Living With Uncertainty 52

Uncertainty Abatement Work 52

Managing Uncertainty 53

Clinical Strategies 54

Case Study 55

CHAPTER **5**

Control 59

Discussion of the Literature 60

Perceived Control 60

Control and Coping 61

Control and Adjustment 61

Illusions of Control 61

The Downside of Control 62

Vicarious Control 62

The Need for Control Is Relative 63

The Need for Control Is Variable 63

Relinquishing Control 64

Clinical Implications 64

Increased Threat: Increased Control 65

Causal Attributions to Regain Control 66

Individualize Interventions to Support Realistic
Personal Control 66

Spectrum of Emotional Reactions 67

When Control Is Needed to Mitigate Distress 67

Control Comes at a Cost 68

Control What You Can 68

Shift in Focus of Control 69

Control-Enhancing Strategies 69

Clinical Strategies 70

Case Study 70

CHAPTER **6**

Suffering 75

Discussion of the Literature 76

What Is Suffering? 76

The Nature of Suffering 76

Isolation 77

Self-Conflict 77

Personal Growth 78

Controlling Suffering: Is it Possible? 78

Individual Interpretation of Suffering 79

Sources of Suffering 79

Chronic Sorrow 80

Clinical Implications 81

The Personal Context of Suffering 81

Caring by Sharing the Suffering of Patients 82

What Do Patients Want From Caregivers? 83

Relieving Suffering 83

Listen From the Heart 83

Compassion 84

Meaning of Suffering 84

Loss of Connection 85

Interventions for Patients With Chronic Sorrow 85

The Suffering of the Family 86

The Suffering of the Staff 87

Clinical Strategies 88

Case Study 88

CHAPTER **7**

Meaning of Illness 93

Discussion of the Literature 94

Personal Meaning 94

The Search for Meaning 94

The Outcome of the Search 95

Personal Meaning and Outcomes 96

Meaning Is Relative 96

Facing Mortality 97

When Meaning Is Negative or Nonexistent 97

Personal Web of Meaning 98

Clinical Implications 98

Personal Meaning of Cancer 99

Personal Meaning as a Dynamic Process 100

Supporting the Discovery of Personal Meaning 101

Authentic Presence 101

Personal Stories 102

Grief Work 103

Supporting Meaningful Connections 103

Unconditional Personal Worth and Value 104

Use of Avoidance Strategies 104

Our Clinical Reality 105

The Need for Personal Reflection 105

    Clinical Strategies 106

    Case Study 106

CHAPTER 8

Forgiveness 111

Discussion of the Literature 112

    An Integrated Concept of Forgiveness 112

    Individual Differences in Forgiveness 113

    What Is Forgiveness? 113

    Forgiveness as a Therapeutic Event 113

    Self-Forgiveness 114

    Forgiveness in Situations of Illness 114

Clinical Implications 115

    Assessing the Need for Forgiveness 115

    The Process of Forgiving 116

    Attribution Retraining 117

    Conflict Resolution 117

The Reciprocal Nature of Forgiveness 118

Anticipating Conflicts 118

Correcting Misconceptions 118

Supporting the Work of Forgiveness 119

Our Contributions to Support Forgiveness 119

The Violation of Illness 119

Clinical Strategies 120

Case Study 121

CHAPTER **9**

Overview of Assessment and Management Strategies 125

Assessment of Depressive Symptomatology 126

Developing a Treatment Plan 127

Risk Factors for Depression 128

Major Depressive Episode 128

Management Issues 129

Treatment of Major Depression 129

Assessment of Anxiety 130

Risk Factors 130

Management Issues 131

General Counseling Interventions 131

Some Thoughts on Compassion 132

Humility 133

APPENDIX **A**

General Interventions, According to Life Stage, to be Used as a Guide for Clinicians 136

APPENDIX **B**

Relaxation and Meditation Practices 142

Index 147

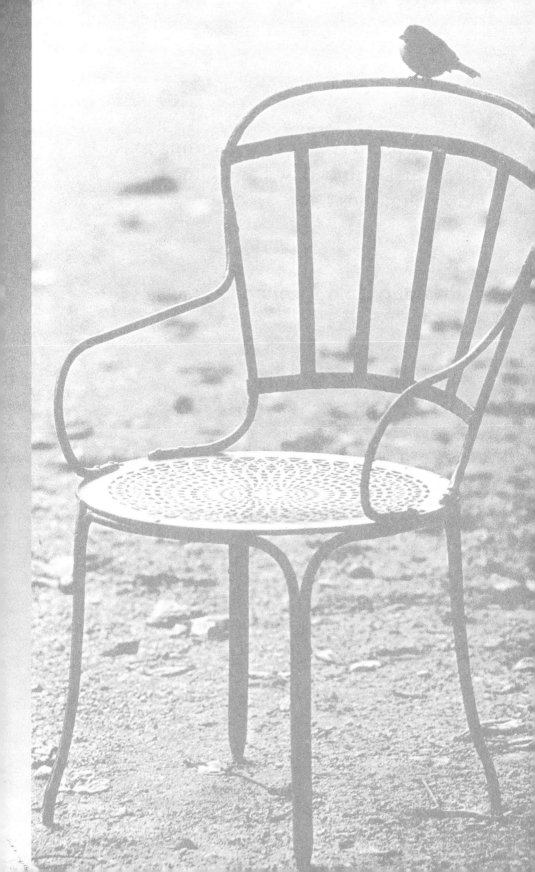

CHAPTER 1

Where's the "Magic Bullet"?

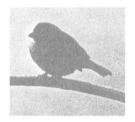

"The day I found out I had cancer I felt like a bomb exploded in my life. It shattered my old life to pieces. I didn't know what I should do or where I should go from there. I no longer had control over my life."

DISCUSSION OF THE LITERATURE

A diagnosis of cancer can derail an individual's life. As Holland (1995) notes, cancer can shake the equanimity of the strongest individual. The emotional distress and turmoil triggered by a cancer diagnosis or recurrence may cause such intense psychological pain that many patients search for immediate relief to control the upset. While acknowledging how painful this distress can be for our patients, as oncology clinicians, we must help them understand that this distress is normal and adaptive. Indeed, psychological distress is not a sign of personal weakness. Patients need to understand further that their own natural style of coping is the best way to cope with their illness.

AVOIDING THE COOKBOOK RECIPES

Beware of the purported magic bullet. It is only an illusion. There are many "cookbook recipes" available for those who are coping with cancer that are designed to provide quick relief. These strategies may work for some, at least for a brief period of time; however, for others, they only create further distress, particularly for those whose personal coping styles don't match the proscribed recipe. Moreover, admonitions and advice from well-meaning friends and family members on how to "positively cope" may add to the search for simple solutions. This often well-intentioned advice may take the form of demands that the cancer patient must be the exceptional patient—one who is unwaveringly positive, always fighting the disease, never showing any negative emotion. The patient may feel the need to "keep a stiff upper lip," to control and to conceal all emotions.

If distress is expressed, it may be interpreted that the patient is "giving up the battle" or "allowing negative emotions to further weaken the immune system and cause the disease to spread." These judgments only create additional stress for the patient and may place strain on significant relationships. The disease, its treatment, and the subsequent psychological distress all converge to put the patient in a vulnerable position, prone to self-doubt. Patients may question the efficacy of their own coping abilities and judgments. Thus, at a time when people with cancer need support and validation of their feelings, unreasonable demands, self-imposed or other-imposed, may interfere with adaptive coping.

The fundamental problem with this line of thinking is that the exceptional patient is fictional. Psychological distress is a normal human reaction to the crisis of a cancer diagnosis or recurrence and is to be expected. In response to this distress, there is no one correct coping style. Clearly, it's not just life as usual.

UPSET IS EXPECTED

A major life crisis has occurred, and a stress reaction follows. In their seminal work, Weisman and Worden (1976–1977, p. 3) describe the initial response to a cancer diagnosis as an "existential plight," which includes fear of abandonment, loss of control, loneliness, and psychological pain. Subsequent research and clinical work support these findings, reaffirming that cancer is a stressful life event that evokes distress as a matter of course. This upset is a necessary and expected part of the emotional adjustment to a significant life crisis. How distress is manifested, its intensity, and duration vary among patients and depend on many factors, such as site and stage of illness, prognosis, age, developmental level, coping style, available support, and concurrent stressors (Rowland, 1989).

RESPONSE PHASES

There are some common themes of psychological response over time as adaptation occurs, with individual variations in the degree and type of distress expressed. In general, there is expected to be a three-phase response to the cancer diagnosis or recurrence (Massie & Holland, 1989). Phase one consists of shock, disbelief, and denial. Many patients describe feeling emotionally detached and socially disconnected as if "they are walking through a bad dream" completely alone. "Life is going on for others but not for me."

Phase two consists of anxiety, depressed mood, anger, guilt, poor concentration, appetite, and sleep problems. During this phase, some patients search for reasons for the illness to make sense of the situation. Some patients may struggle with the question, "Why me?" While others ask, "Why not me?" Last, phase three includes adjustment to illness and treatment demands. During this phase, the challenge is to come to terms with the realities of the illness and treatment, while incorporating necessary changes into daily life.

These phases are not necessarily sequential or self-contained; thus, some patients may experience a combination of denial, upset, and adjustment in rapid succession. Others may experience one phase predominately. Also, the timetable for these expected responses varies significantly. For example, some patients remain "numb" and emotionally detached until after adjuvant treatment is completed. It's important to understand that each patient will have a unique emotional response.

Similarly, it is important to let patients know that this psychological distress is expected and may occur at various points either during treatment or after its completion. Emotional distress is necessary and adaptive. It signals the need for the requisite cognitive and emotional processing of this significant life event, and it provides the opportunity to make necessary life changes and realign priorities to adapt to the changes necessitated by the disease and its treatment. However, if the emotional reactions become intense, disruptive, and persistent, interfering with daily living and interpersonal relationships, patients should be referred for psychological evaluation (see Chap. 9).

In summary, distress is a normal part of the adjustment process. It should be anticipated rather than criticized or denied, and a system of support must be put in place, guided by the individual patient's needs and coping style.

MIND AND BODY WORK

There are those who argue against this normal stress response. The mind–body literature is often used as evidence to support the premise that people with cancer are "harming their immune systems" if they experience upsetting thoughts or feelings. Because mind–body work tends to be highly publicized, the potential easily exists for misinterpretation of unconfirmed data (Holland, 1991).

Currently, scientific data from mind–body studies are preliminary and contradictory and do not support the notion that the distress associated with a cancer diagnosis exacerbates cancer or that stress causes cancer. Moreover, the complex interactions of the brain, neuroendocrine system, and immune system make these issues highly complex and difficult to sort out.

The field of mind–body study or psychoneuroimmunology (PNI) has its origins in psychosomatic medicine and has evolved into the investigation of complex interactions between the psyche and the nervous, immune, and endocrine systems (Fife, Beasley, & Fertig, 1996).

PSYCHONEUROIMMUNOLOGY RESEARCH FINDINGS

To date, the psychological factors studied are mostly short-term effects of emotions on neuroendocrine or immune function under experimental and clinical circumstances (Dantzer, 1997). These emotions have been shown to influence a number of different physiological responses, but mechanisms of action and the clinical meaning of these neuroimmunological changes still await further study (Bovbjerg, 1991). While significant associations have been found between stressful life events and neuroimmune changes, a causal link among stress, immune function, and disease has not been established. However, major links between these systems are being described, and PNI is developing the techniques to explore these interactive relationships and their clinical implications further (Anderson, 1996).

With more sophisticated techniques, there are many promising studies certain to elucidate our understanding of the complex mind–body connections. What we do know is that patients should not be blamed for their normal emotional responses of worry and concern no matter how these may be expressed.

PSYCHONEUROIMMUNOLOGY AND CANCER

Specific to PNI and cancer, Fox (1995) critically reviewed the relationships between psychological variables and the presence of cancer, its prediction, and the prediction of cancer mortality and the course of disease. He noted for the psychological variables most intensely studied, such as depressed mood; suppression of emotions, especially anger, helplessness, and hopelessness; and social support, the literature remains contradictory. That is, studies have shown both positive relationships and absence of relationships.

Fox (1995) goes on to note various research problems with methodology and design in the mind–body literature that obscure accurate findings. He concludes that in answer to the basic question of possible influence of psychological factors on cancer, it seems fairly certain that the influence ranges from no or little influence to uncertain influence at best. Some people under certain conditions for some cancer types may be affected by psychological factors, for example, more aggressive disease. However, much remains to be understood about the mechanism of action.

WHAT DO THE FINDINGS MEAN?

These findings should not be seen as negating the importance of psychological states, but rather, cautioning us not to overstate the existing scientific evidence and imply disease causation or disease progression. While there are no definitive answers about psychological states and their link to illnesses such as cancer, the data are unquestioned that psychological factors are strong determinants of behavior and have a significant impact on adaptive coping and quality of life (Holland, 1995).

What can we apply from PNI to guide clinical practice? There is clear evidence that stressors have significant influence on neuroimmune responses, but different perceptions of stress result in different patterns of neuroendocrine activation (Dantzer, 1997; Henry, 1992) with different physiological consequences. The psychological nature of the stressor, in particular the person's ability to control and predict its occurrence, is more important than its physical nature (Henry & Wang, 1998). As Ursin (1998) states, we have known for over 30 years that psychological influences are among the most powerful natural stimuli known to affect pituitary-adrenal cortical activity. Particularly potent influences on the system are novelty, uncertainty, and unpredictability. There are marked differences in individual responses to any particular situation dependent on multiple psychological and physiological determinants.

Thus, there are some valuable clinical implications from PNI research that can guide clinical practice. Of particular importance are those strategies that enhance control, reduce uncertainty, and elucidate understanding of the individual's perception of the illness and its meaning.

CLINICAL IMPLICATIONS

Cancer is an unpredictable and uncertain disease that can create heightened vulnerability for many patients. The scientific research to date supports the importance of understanding the personal meaning of the illness to our patients, enhancing control, and offering patients support that is congruent with their manner of coping style.

As health professionals, what can we do to provide support for patients and families who are coping with cancer-related distress? The goal of psychosocial oncology care is to understand the unique needs and strengths of the patient and family to create an individualized plan of care that promotes optimal psychological adaptation (Houldin & Lowery, 1992). Perhaps the best way to offer this support is understanding our patients' perceptions of their illness and matching supportive interventions to their personal coping style.

ANSWERING COMMON QUESTIONS

A number of common questions from patients and family members should be anticipated:

- Should patients with cancer be encouraged to verbalize their feelings?
- Should they be told to avoid denial?
- Should they remain positive, hopeful, and maintain a fighting spirit?
- Will they cause harm to themselves if they feel upset?
- How do they regain control?

We must tell our patients that there is *no one right way to cope*! Each person needs to find what works for him or her within the context of accepted oncology practice. Understandably, during this time of turmoil, many patients want to be told what to do. We can tell them the following: (1) trust their innate coping skills; (2) they should not be blamed for their disease or for their upset; (3) it is not a sign of weakness to express distress; (4) have confidence in their own judgments; and (5) take control of lowering stressors in their lives and enhance personal support.

THE PERCEPTIONS OF OUR PATIENTS

We need to understand what this illness means to our patients and take time to get to know our patients' beliefs and values. The psychological issues are complex and are influenced by many variables, such as personality style, personal values and goals, maturity level, individual perception and personal meaning of the illness, past experiences with illness or loss, and availability of support. We need to appreciate the fact that individuals' responses to illness reflect their long-standing approach to life.

NORMALIZE DISTRESS

It's important to understand our patients' distress without pressure to have all the answers. We must give our patients and their family members permission to experience the upset as normal and as an important first step in the healing process. We need to inform patients that emotional pain will not last forever as is commonly feared. The distress is necessary to experience to come to terms with the realities and demands of the disease. We must assist patients to regain control and reduce uncertainty. Some strategies that are helpful in achieving these goals include:

- Explaining normal psychological responses to illness
- Informing patients about support groups and community resources
- Providing information about side effects of medications and treatments
- Explaining diagnostic tests, interpreting results, and teaching symptom management

THE DISTRESS OF LOVED ONES

We need to acknowledge the strain on family members, offering validation of their feelings and their right to experience upset even though they are not ill. We must be ready to help the patient and family navigate through the cancer experience, with the clear realization that cancer is a family illness and that each person who is emotionally connected to the patient is experiencing distress. This can be accomplished by putting support in place for significant others. Offering guidance that the best support the family can offer a patient is to "be there" emotionally for their loved one by allowing the individual to express emotions without judgment or criticism. Perhaps learning to respect personal feelings and asking for and accepting support is the best advice we can give both patients and their significant others.

CONTRADICTING INFORMATION

Because of increasing public information and the potential for misuse of the mind–body data, patients should be informed about the contradictory and preliminary state of PNI research. They should know that the available data do not support notions about one correct intervention or one right attitude. A "fighting spirit" or a "positive attitude" does not cure cancer! The current state of the science suggests there are many healthy ways of coping with illness (Lowery & Houldin, 1996). We must empower our patients to use their own innate coping skills. Discover what has worked for patients during previous life crises, and encourage them to put those strategies in place now.

In summary, it is important to

- Teach both patients and their loved ones about the normal stress response.
- Help them to anticipate the nature and course of the expected distress.
- Debunk myths related to expressing upset.
- Support both patients and family members.
- Enhance personal control.
- Encourage respect for individual coping style differences.

CLINICAL STRATEGIES

1. Assess the patient's emotional state, and identify the primary concerns. Some pertinent assessment questions are as follows: What is the meaning of this illness to you? What are the most pressing problems? What are your goals? How can we help?
2. Respect the patient's uniqueness, and use skills of active listening to understand the patient's coping skills. What has worked well for the patient during times of crisis? What is the patient's usual coping style?

3. Combine common sense, sensitivity, empathy, and compassion with knowledge of the patient's needs and resources.
4. Advise patients not to waste time and energy searching for the "right way" to cope.
5. Validate the normalcy and healing function of distress.
6. Reaffirm personal control by telling patients to use the coping skills that work best for them.
7. Encourage patients to communicate their feelings and to ask for what they need from others.
8. Offer support to family members and significant others. Encourage them to understand and respect coping differences. Let them know that they aren't expected to have all the answers. Their most helpful response is simply to listen.
9. Distress is not a sign of weakness, and seeking personal support is a sign of strength. Acknowledge the distress, and give patients and loved ones permission to experience it.

CASE STUDY

CM, a 52-year-old married woman and mother of three adult children, was diagnosed with advanced colorectal cancer. She had an established career and was well-respected for her many professional contributions. CM enjoyed good health until this unexpected diagnosis following a bout of abdominal distress. Following extensive abdominal surgery for her disease, she was recuperating at home before beginning a recommended course of chemotherapy. During this time, CM had episodes of crying, increased worry and nervousness, and difficulty sleeping. Given that CM was a very stoic individual who rarely displayed any emotion before her illness, this upset was a matter of great concern to her and her family. In addition, she began to complain of increasing fatigue, poor appetite, nausea, and significant abdominal pain that intensified rather than diminished, as one would expect as she recuperated from surgery. Her family attributed these symptoms to her psychological distress that, if unabated, would weaken her ability to fight the disease and to "beat the cancer."

Her husband and children searched the Internet and local book stores for mind–body information and encouraged CM to read all the information they could find on alternative therapy and "mind–body" healing. As much as she tried the various techniques, positive thinking, imagery, and so on, CM was not able to rid herself of these problems; in fact, the symptoms intensified to the point of her becoming housebound and barely able to get out of bed during the day. In desperation, CM called a local oncology counselor to inquire about what else she could do to rid herself of this psychological turmoil, inability to "think positively," and the constant worry that she was killing herself because of her "lousy attitude." CM requested an antidepressant. Fortunately, upon hearing of the intensity and duration of the symptoms, the counselor recommended that CM contact her surgeon immediately to report these significant problems. That same day, CM was admitted to the hospital and found to be suffering from a complication that required immediate surgical intervention.

This case study illustrates potential dangers of the exaggerated and well-publicized "benefits" of mind–body healing techniques. CM and her family were frightened. They were used to exercising a great deal of control in their daily lives. When the cancer diagnosis struck "the pillar of strength in their family" so unexpectedly, they were devastated. Everyone scrambled to regain control of the situation. The family latched on to mind-control techniques as something that could benefit their loved one, but in the frantic process of trying to fix the problem, they overlooked the obvious with potentially disastrous consequences.

REFERENCES

Anderson, J. L. (1996). The immune system and major depression. *Advances in Neuroimmunology, 6*(2), 119–129.

Bovbjerg, D. H. (1991, February 1). Psychoneuroimmunology: What are the implications for oncology? *Cancer, 67*(Suppl. 3), 828–832.

Dantzer, R. (1997). Stress and immunity: What have we learned from psychoneuroimmunology? *Acta Physiologica Scandinavia Supplementum, 640,* 43–46.

Fife, A., Beasley, P. J., & Fertig, D. L. (1996). Psychoneuroimmunology and cancer: Historical perspectives and current research. *Advances in Neuroimmunology, 6*(2), 179–190.

Fox, B. H. (1995). The role of psychological factors in cancer incidence and prognosis. *Oncology, March 9*(3), 245–255.

Henry, J. P. (1992). Biological basis of the stress response. *Integrative Physiological and Behavioral Science, 27,* 66–83.

Henry, J. P., & Wang, S. (1998). Effects of early stress on adult affiliative behavior. *Psychoneuroendocrinology, 23*(8), 863–875.

Holland, J. C. (1991, October). *Psychosocial variables: Are they factors in cancer risk or survival?* Paper presented at Current Concepts in Psych-Oncology conference cosponsored by Memorial Sloan-Kettering Cancer Center, European School of Oncology, and International Psycho-Oncology Society, New York.

Holland, J. C. (1995). The role of psychological factors in cancer incidence and prognosis: Article review. *Oncology, March 9*(3), 256.

Houldin, A. D., & Lowery, B. J. (1992). Emotional distress in breast cancer patients. *Med-Surg Nursing Quarterly, 1*(2), 1–28.

Lowery, B. J., & Houldin, A. D. (1996). From stressor to illness: The psychological-biological connections. In A. McBride & J. Austin (Eds.), *Psychiatric-mental health nursing: Integrating the behavioral and biological sciences* (pp. 11–29). Philadelphia: W.B. Saunders.

Massie, M. J., & Holland, J. C. (1989). Overview of normal reactions and prevalence of psychiatric disorders. In Holland J. C. & Rowland, J. H. (Eds.), *Handbook of psychooncology* (pp. 273–290). New York: Oxford University Press.

Rowland, J. H. (1989). Intrapersonal resources: Coping. In Holland J. C. & Rowland, J. H. (Eds.), *Handbook of psychooncology* (pp. 44–57). New York: Oxford University Press.

Ursin, H. (1998). The psychology in psychoneuroendocrinology. *Psychoneuroendocrinology, August 23*(6), 555–570.

Weisman, A. D., & Worden, C. B. (1976–1977). The existential plight in cancer: Significance of the first 100 days. *International Journal of Psychiatry in Medicine, 7*(1), 1–15.

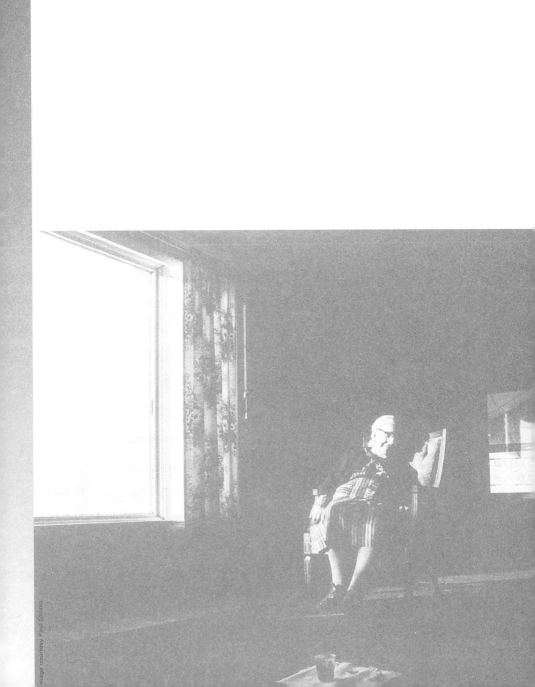

CHAPTER 2

Denial

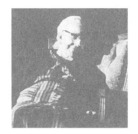

"Denial is not my choice. It is my obligation. It's expected by my family, my friends, and even by my doctor. If I talk about how sick I am and how worried I am about dying, I'm told that I'm letting those who love me down. I'm hurting them with my negativity. I'm losing hope. It makes it easier for them if I pretend. So I do."

DISCUSSION OF THE LITERATURE

A central question in oncology practice today is how to balance the reality of the illness with reasonable hope.

Thinking on denial has come full circle, from early psychoanalytic teaching that denial was maladaptive, an immature defense to be confronted (Fenichel, 1978), to later understanding that denial was an adaptive response to illness (Lazarus, 1983). Currently, denial is more likely to be promoted, implicitly or explicitly, to avoid confronting the reality of life-threatening illness (Ross, Peteet, Medeiros, Walsh-Burke, & Rieker, 1992)

Today, a challenge in oncology practice is not so much the confrontation of denial, but rather the avoidance of collusion with its use. Influenced by popular social thinking about the virtues of positive thinking and the need to maintain hope despite all odds, denial has become a mainstay for many patients, families, and even professional staff. Adding urgency to this movement is the suggestion that denial may even be associated with prolonged survival, at least for some cancer patients (Greer, 1992). Thus, in current practice, there is significant public pressure on oncology staff, particularly physicians, to maintain hope and avoid negativity regardless of the medical reality.

WHAT IS DENIAL?

Denial is a complex concept that has different meanings in different contexts and serves a multitude of functions. For patients coping with physical illness, denial is often viewed as a strategy used by emotionally healthy people in stressful circumstances (Ness & Ende, 1994). Denial, in these situations, provides psychological protection against the perception and processing of painful or distressing information (Goldbeck, 1997). As such, denial is considered an early reaction to cancer diagnosis or recurrence and is subsequently replaced by other coping responses (Massie & Holland, 1989). However, denial of the illness or of its severity for some can cause delayed diagnosis or compromise compliance with treatment (Kunkel, Woods, Rodgers, & Myers, 1997; Zervas, Augustine, & Fricchione, 1993). Furthermore, denial is used within an interpersonal context. Each person determines what information can be shared with others (Ross et al., 1992). Thus, some patients may use denial to preserve relationships of importance to them (Weisman, 1972; Connor, 1992), which may compromise their ability to communicate honestly their concerns and fears and receive the necessary support. The level of denial among family members may also influence denial on the patient's part (Ness & Ende, 1994).

DENIAL IN FAMILY MEMBERS

For family members, distressed by the news of their loved one's illness, denial is often used at least initially as a self-protective strategy while coming to terms with the impact of the diagnosis. Some family members have the added burden of the perceived need to "protect" the patient from upsetting information and the loss of hope, which may in turn reinforce denial in themselves and in the patient. On the other hand, there are those who view denial as problematic and feel the need to confront any sign of denial in the patient. Perhaps by focusing on patient denial, some family members are better able to distract themselves from their own fear and vulnerability and exert some measure of control over the situation.

DENIAL IN STAFF

For oncology staff, a similar range of possible reactions exists. There are those who need to encourage patient denial for self-protective reasons shaped in part by their own needs to avoid emotions associated with mortality (Ross et al., 1992); those who need to confront denial, viewing it as maladaptive; and those who can balance the need for accurate, honest information with a supportive, hopeful approach. Many oncology clinicians appear to fall in this last category.

Ross et al. (1992) reported that the majority of cancer center physicians and nurses they studied viewed denial as an adaptive coping mechanism but recognized that denial can interfere with realistic planning and may require individualized attempts at modification. However, these investigators also found that physicians often expressed willingness to allow or even support denial for patients and families more frequently than nurses did. In some cases, the need to maintain patients' hope seemed to override other medical considerations and goals. The nurses' goal was to avoid promoting patients' denial because of concerns about futile treatments, lack of awareness of the nearness of death, and patients not being able to complete the business of their lives.

Thus, while there may be discipline-related differences in response to patient denial, clearly there are individual differences as well.

It is important for all clinicians to understand their contribution to denial to ensure that the patient receives factual, clear information regarding the disease and its implications. As Ross et al. (1992) note, wide variation in a patient's handling of information may be acceptable as long as the patient is receiving the facts necessary to make an informed decision.

DENIAL: PROCESS AND OUTCOMES

Goldbeck (1997), in a comprehensive review of denial in physical illness, provides some important insights on denial as a process. He summarizes that denial is not an all or nothing phenomenon, but is expressed along a continuum of behaviors. Denial is a dynamic process with temporal fluctuations and situational factors influencing its expression. For example, denial may represent the early stages of an adaptational process or may emerge during times of particular stress.

Outcomes research on denial has produced mixed results. Overall for patients with physical illness, denial may have some positive mood-regulating effects (Goldbeck, 1997). However, results concerning the relationship between denial and medical outcomes have been conflicting and inconclusive. Some empirical studies suggest that denial may serve a useful purpose early on but may become maladaptive if sustained over prolonged periods of time (Levine et al., 1987). Other studies note the association between denial and diagnostic delays and treatment noncompliance (Kunkel, Woods, Rodgers, & Myers, 1997).

DENIAL IN PATIENTS

Lazarus (1983) proposes some guiding principles to help determine if patient denial is adaptive:

1. A careful assessment of each person's circumstances. If denial inhibits action of importance, for example, compliance with treatment, then it may be regarded as maladaptive; however, if it is experienced in the face of an unalterable situation, it may afford comfort and enhance coping.
2. While denial may have advantages during the early stages following a distressing event, it may prevent appropriate adaptation if sustained over extended periods of time.
3. Distinguish between a fact being denied (eg, diagnosis of cancer) and implications of the fact denied (eg, cancer will not return). The former may interfere with necessary treatment; the latter may maintain morale in a difficult situation.
4. Does denial enhance the patient's ability to interpret events in a positive manner?

In summary, denial is a mechanism used for psychological protection. It provides benefit for some individuals in certain circumstances. However, for others, it may interfere with treatment decisions, communication, and appropriate planning. Further, it is important to understand denial in a broad context. Specifically, what is the purpose and function of denial for the patient, family, and staff? Denial must be understood within the personal as well as interpersonal and social contexts.

CLINICAL IMPLICATIONS

Denial is a self-protective response used to lower distress when individuals feel overwhelmed and threatened. It is an important and necessary phase when adapting to the realities of a serious illness. The use of and need for denial will fluctuate over time and will likely be intensified at critical points in the disease trajectory. As such, we need to understand denial and its unique purpose for each of our patients over the course of the illness.

ASSESSING DENIAL

Carefully consider denial; for example, how and when it is used by the patient, the benefits and risks, the patient's usual coping style, the function it serves within the family unit, and its purpose for the patient and for others. Denial may be expressed in various ways, such as downward comparison, minimization of illness, or lack of emotional response. If these responses are present, it signals that the patient is frightened. Rather than confronting denial or challenging assumptions, it's best to provide support for patients to discuss issues of concern as they are able and at their own pace.

When denial compromises patients' safety, it must be addressed directly. Some common situations include patients not reporting symptoms or not following through with prescribed medication or recommended medical care. Also, when denial inhibits actions of importance, for example, interference with informed treatment decision making, ability to plan realistically, and honest communication with loved ones, it is also important to intervene.

WHEN DENIAL CAUSES PROBLEMS

If denial is causing significant problems, direct confrontation may only increase the use of denial. Nonconfrontational techniques, for example, providing factual information, using a nonjudgmental approach, listening empathetically, reflecting, summarizing, and problem-solving, are helpful interventions (Miller, 1983; Ness & Ende, 1994). Ness & Ende (1994) note that the aim in these cases should be to find the best strategy for helping the patient overcome the fearfulness that stands in the way of accepting the reality of the illness. These authors recommend using surface approaches as opposed to depth approaches to enhance patient control and reduce fearfulness. That is, focus on the specific symptom or problem rather than on the more central need for denial. For example, encourage a patient to use pain medications to increase independence and control over symptoms. In this way, the need for control is acknowledged, but the denial of the meaning of pain is not confronted directly. Further, if a patient's need for denial interferes with accurate reporting of symptoms, it may be necessary to identify a reliable family member to accompany the patient to medical visits to provide the necessary information. Thus, it is important to recognize when patient denial is interfering with treatment, ensure that care is not compromised, and offer support and understanding while addressing patients' denial using nonconfrontational strategies.

PERCEPTION OF DENIAL

It is important to understand that denial is an interpreted phenomenon (Shelp & Perl, 1985). The interpretation of denial by others is clearly influenced by their own views and biases. Thus, in the interpretation of clinicians, what appears to be patient denial may in fact be lack of information, lack of understanding, or lack of agreement with medical recommendations (Cousins, 1982; Shelp & Perl, 1985). Similarly, when significant others worry that the patient is not upset enough or is minimizing the implications of the illness, the concerns may reflect their own needs and issues rather than those of the patient. In these situations, it's important to assess our own and family members' biases, fears, and concerns and to offer support and education about the utility of denial and the dangers of direct confrontation. As clinicians, we must carefully assess our patients' reasoning driving their behavior and responses before reaching conclusions.

We may also need to help patients set limits when others attempt to confront them with what they perceive as patient denial. For example, limiting the disclosure of detailed medical information, pointing out that the patient does not want to discuss the illness repeatedly when socializing, and reminding family members that patients should set the tone and control the depth and content of discussions about their illness.

WHEN DENIAL PROTECTS OTHERS

In some instances, patients use denial not to protect themselves, but to protect family members who are not ready to confront the realities of the illness. Thus, it is important to understand the motivation for the use of denial. It is useful to observe family dynamics during visits. Are family members able to allow patients to discuss concerns and fears without cutting them off, admonishing them, or cheering them up? Do family members express concern that the patient is too negative or not hopeful enough? The following interventions may be helpful in these situations:

1. Educating the patient and significant others on the importance of keeping lines of communication open
2. Validating the normalcy of worry and distress for both patient and family

3. Assessing level of anxiety and distress in family members
4. Making referrals to counseling or support groups

PROMOTING DENIAL

As clinicians, we need to be aware of the pitfalls of colluding with patient or family denial. As Stewart (1994) notes, medical staff may promote denial in patients by failing to explain fully the nature or extent of disease or by not probing enough for possible denial (Ness & Ende, 1994). Denial may be used for the purpose of protecting staff or as a response to external pressures to be hopeful and positive. We need to reflect on our own motivations and approaches to disclosing medical information to patients. Are we contributing overtly or covertly to patient denial? Whose needs are being met by the use of denial? The use of denial ought to be driven by the needs of the patient, not by the needs of the staff.

WHEN DENIAL INTERFERES WITH COMMUNICATION

Although we can't regulate the need for denial in our patients, we can communicate facts related to the disease and its treatment unambiguously and repeatedly. When bad news must be given, we should be prepared to spend additional time to provide emotional support to patients and families. Patients need to understand that the medical goal is to present factual information in an understandable manner so that patients can make fully informed decisions about care. We must also educate patients and families about the downside to denial. Denial can isolate patients from loved ones when they desperately need their support. If patients and families don't have a realistic understanding of the disease and its likely implications, it limits informed decision making and robs them of precious time to make wishes known and put business and personal matters in order. Denial particularly may hurt children by isolating them and not allowing them to participate in the decision-making process.

CLINICAL STRATEGIES

1. Assess the nature, purpose, and function of denial at various times across the disease trajectory. Some assessment questions are as follows:
   A. Is the patient denying the fact of the illness or its implications?
   B. What is the evidence to support the use of denial?
   C. What effect is denial having on patient behavior?
   D. What is the effect on relationships with others, including the medical team?
   E. How is the patient's denial expressed?
   F. Are there harmful consequences of the patient's use of denial? If so, what are they?
   G. What are the benefits of using denial?
   M. What purpose is denial serving?
   I. Is it being used for the protection of others?
2. When denial interferes with the management of the illness or the well-being of the patient, it should be thoughtfully and sensitively addressed using nonconfrontational techniques.
3. It is important to help family members sort out reasons for either their need for denial or excessive focus on patient denial.
4. Clinicians need to understand their need for or contribution to the use of denial. Sort out personal needs and external pressures that may interfere with presenting a realistic view of the disease and its implications.
5. Unequivocally, patients need to be informed clearly, fully, and supportively about their diagnosis and prognosis. How they are told and in what detail are functions of numerous factors related to the patient, family, and medical team. These interactions cannot be proscribed, but it is important for clinicians to set the tone for frank and open discussions early in the disease course.
6. Emphasize to patients that they will not be abandoned. They will be supported and cared for, whether the medical news is good or bad.

CASE STUDY

CG was a 72-year-old woman recently diagnosed with pancreatic cancer. At the time of diagnosis, her husband of 50 years was quite ill with a cardiac problem. She had two adult children. Both were very involved in their par-

Continued

ents' care. CG was a positive, cheerful patient who held much hope for a complete recovery. She was also a religious person who took great comfort from her spiritual beliefs. The patient and her family were fully informed in a frank but supportive manner as to the illness, its treatment, and prognosis. As CG began chemotherapy, her children approached the oncology staff with the fear that their mother was not "being realistic." She was too positive and hopeful. She had not cried or expressed any visible upset. They feared CG would be devastated when the illness progressed. The staff encouraged the family to allow the patient to adjust to the diagnosis and treatment on her own terms. They pointed out how overwhelming the illness, coupled with her husband's frail condition, was to the patient. The staff pointed out that CG was an intelligent woman who understood the implications of her disease and predicted that when the patient was ready to deal with the emotional aspects of her illness, she would. CG was referred to counseling and began keeping a journal of her thoughts and feelings. Gradually and in a controlled manner, CG was able to express her distress and worry about her and her husband's illnesses and the possible outcomes. She remained hopeful and comforted by her spiritual beliefs. Her children, who were also seen in separate counseling sessions, were able to understand their motivation to focus on their mother's denial as a focal point to avoid facing their own pain and grief.

REFERENCES

Connor, S. R. (1992). Denial in terminal illness: to intervene or not to intervene. *Hospice Journal, 8*(4), 1–15.

Cousins, N. (1982). Denial: Are sharper definitions needed? *Journal of the American Medical Association, 248,* 210–212.

Fenichel, O. (1978). *The psychoanalytic theory of neurosis.* London: Routledge & Kegan Paul.

Goldbeck, R. (1997). Denial in physical illness. *Journal of Psychosomatic Research, 43*(6), 575–593.

Greer, S. (1992). The management of denial in cancer patients. *Oncology, 6*(12), 33–40.

Kunkel, E. J., Woods, C. M., Rodgers, C., & Myers, R. E. (1997). Consultations for maladaptive denial of illness in patients with cancer: Psychiatric disorders that result in noncompliance. *Psycho-Oncology, 6*(2), 139-149.

Lazarus, R. S. (1983). The costs and benefits of denial. In Breznitz, S. (Ed.), *The denial of stress* (pp. 3–30). New York: International University Press.

Levine, J., Warrenburg, S., Kerns, R., Schwartz, G., Delaney, R., Fontana, A., Gradman, A., Smith, S., Allen, S., & Cascione, R. (1987). The role of denial in recovery from coronary heart disease. *Psychosomatic Medicine, 49*(2), 109–117.

Massie, M. J., & Holland, J. C. (1989). Overview of normal reactions and prevalence of psychiatric disorders. In J. C. Holland, & J. H. Rowland (Eds.), *Handbook of psychooncology* (pp. 273–282). New York: Oxford University Press.

Miller, W. R. (1983). Motivational interviewing with problem drinkers. *Behavioral Psychotherapeutics, 11,* 147–172.

Ness, D. E., & Ende, J. (1994). Denial in the medical interview. *Journal of the American Medical Association, 273,* 1777–1781.

Ross, D. M., Peteet, J. R., Medeiros, C., Walsh-Burke, K., & Rieker, P. (1992). Difference between nurses' and physicians' approach to denial in oncology. *Cancer Nursing, 15*(6), 422–428.

Shelp E. E., & Perl, M. (1985). Denial in clinical medicine: A reexamination of the concept and its significance. *Archives of Internal Medicine, 145,* 697–699.

Stewart, J. R. (1994). Denial of disabling conditions and specific interventions in the rehabilitation counseling setting. *Journal of Applied Rehabilitation Counseling, 25,* 7–15.

Weisman, A. D. (1972). *On dying and denying: A psychiatric study of terminality.* New York: Behavioral Publications.

Zervas, I. M., Augustine, A., & Fricchione, G. L. (1993). Patient delay in cancer. A view from the crisis model. *General Hospital Psychiatry, 15*(1), 9–13.

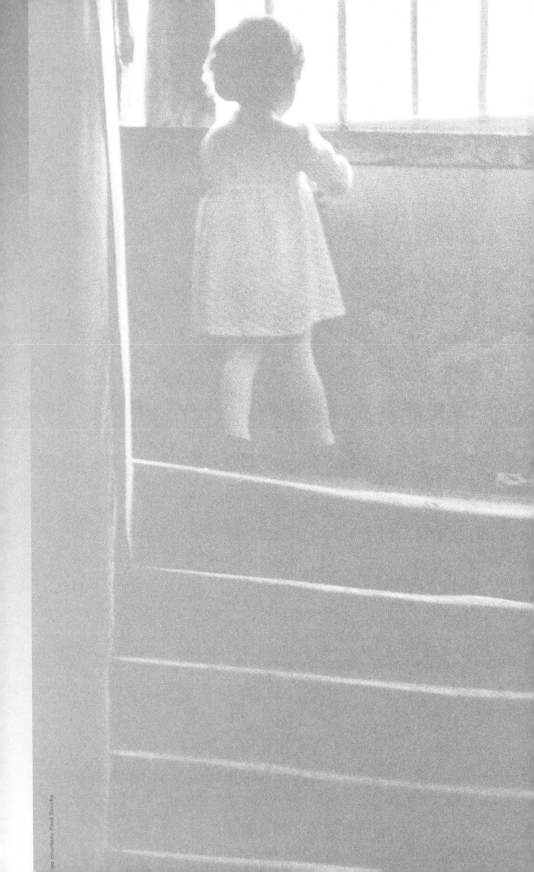

CHAPTER 3

Hope

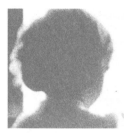

"*Hope deferred makes the heart sick, but when dreams come true at last, there is life and joy*" (Proverbs 13:12).

"*There is no hope without fear nor fear without hope*" (Spinoza).

"*We never live but expect to live. We are never happy because we are always readying ourselves for our future happiness*" (Pascal).

"*When faced with cancer, a sense of hope can provide meaning, direction, motivation, and a reason for being*" (Post-White et al., 1996).

DISCUSSION OF THE LITERATURE

As the preceding quotes illustrate, there are various ways to view the concept of hope. Hope is one of the most cherished ideas in the western culture (Omer & Rosenbaum, 1997). Hope, as a healing power, has long been valued. Hopeful images are now believed to cure not just apathy and depression, but also poverty and cancer (Omer & Rosenbaum, 1997). Hope has been viewed by some as essential for adaptive coping (Lazarus & Folkman, 1984). Loss of hope is implicated as a major feature of a number of psychiatric disorders (Beck, Steer, Kovacs, & Garrison, 1985). For people with medical illness, hope is viewed as essential to maintain a fighting spirit (Greer, 1992). Some research has found that the degree of hope reported by people with cancer actually increased as signs of disease progression were evident (Herth, 1990). Elizabeth Kübler-Ross (1969) argued that people remained hopeful even when confronted with the knowledge of their impending death.

IS HOPE ALWAYS ADAPTIVE?

Others caution against assuming hope is always adaptive and conversely that despair is maladaptive. Some raise the possibility that hope may at times function paradoxically or that despair in certain situations may be therapeutic (Bennett & Bennett, 1984). For example, Omer and Rosenbaum (1997) argue that hope can be maladaptive as a function of its unlikelihood, when it leads to disparagement of the present, to mindless sacrifices, and to rigid attitudes or behaviors. At such times, individuals may need encouragement to let go of hope, and the "work of despair" may provide benefit. Taken further, Comte-Sponville (1984) argues that the renunciation of hope is a requirement for happiness. We hope for an ideal future because we cling to a romanticized image of the past and in so doing, devalue our present reality. Moreover, in the eastern tradition, there has long been a philosophical view that hope is a significant source of unhappiness. Eastern philosophers have argued that hope goes hand in hand with fear and disappointment; hope creates dependent attachments to objects of desire; and hope stands between us and life (Omer & Rosenbaum, 1997).

Hope has been considered sacred by many, and despair to be avoided, but could it be that there may be value to despair? Is hope in fact essential to adaptive coping, or is hope merely an illusion? Does ignoring reality eventually bring its own reckoning?

DEFINING HOPE

Within the context of medical illness, there are many aspects to consider when examining the concept of hope. Hope is a complex and highly subjective phenomenon. As such, it defies precise definition. The literature suggests that hope is a multidimensional construct that provides comfort while enduring life threats and personal challenges (Hinds, 1984). Hope is composed of a wide range of thoughts, feelings, and actions. Herth (1990) defines hope as an inner power directed toward enrichment of being. When attempting to define hope, the most pervasive theme in the literature is that hope is an expectation of attainment of important goals (Stoner, 1983). In illness, hope has often been linked with cure (Nekolaichuk & Bruera, 1998). Thus, it becomes important to distinguish between a generalized hope (the inner experience of hope) and a particularized hope (for a specific goal or outcome) (Dufault & Martocchio, 1985). Some note that particularized hope or objects of hope should be grounded in reality (Hinds & Martin, 1988). A broad working definition particularly applicable to situations of medical illness is that hope is a multidimensional dynamic life force characterized by a confident yet uncertain expectation of achieving a future good, which, to the hoping person, is realistically possible and personally significant (Dufault & Martocchio, 1985).In sum, hope is an elusive, complex concept that, for the purpose of definition, can be dichotomized into internal aspects and external expectations, objects of hope; in application, however, hope is essentially defined by its meaning to a particular individual in any given circumstance.

THE PERSONAL EXPERIENCE OF HOPE

While some research has examined the descriptive and theoretical aspects of the concept of hope, there is limited research on the outcomes of hope (Bunston,

Mings, Mackie, & Jones, 1995). Theoretically, it appears that many factors influence the development and experience of hope. For some, to be in control may be essential to maintain hope. Hopelessness can occur in response to feelings of helplessness or loss of control (Brockopp, Hayko, Davenport, & Winscott, 1989; Hinds & Martin, 1988). For others, to make sense of what is happening is important. That is, the attribution of meaning to present experience with its implications for the future may be central to the process of hoping (Weiner, 1985). Others view perceived social support as being significant in determining hope. That is, nurturing relationships and interconnectedness with others are important to the maintenance of hope (Herth, 1990; Raleigh, 1992). Finally, spiritual beliefs are viewed as central by many (Ellison, 1983; Frankl, 1984) for their significant role in inspiring and sustaining hope. Spiritual aspects of hope have been defined broadly to include the belief that one's future has a purpose and meaning either through one's inherent worth as an individual or through connections with some greater entity (Spencer, Davidson, & White 1997). Essentially, how an individual's desires, values, and fears become consolidated into goals or objects of hope is a uniquely individual matter (Nunn, 1996).

HOPE IN PATIENTS WITH CANCER

The cancer literature generally supports the value and necessity of hope, particularly internal sources of hope, for the most part irrespective of course of the disease (Ersek, 1992; Herth, 1990). As Ballard, Green, McCaa, and Logsdon (1997) note, "the essence of hope gives the patient a tomorrow to look forward to—the possibility that cancer would be cured and life would move on" (p. 900). Post-White et al. (1996) describe five central themes influencing hope for cancer patients: finding meaning, relying on inner resources, affirming relationships, living in the present, and anticipating survival. These investigators also found significant individual variability in defining hope. In addition, Ballard et al. found that patients with newly diagnosed and recurrent cancer did not differ in levels of hope but differed in type of hope. That is, patients experiencing a recurrence tended to emphasize faith as a source of hope, while the newly diagnosed patients focused on hope from health care professionals. Others (Mahon, Cella, & Donovan, 1990) have found that patients with recurrent disease were less hopeful. In terms of patient outcomes, there is some evidence that hope may enhance adjustment to illness (Christ-man, 1990; Ersek, 1992) and contribute to improved quality of life (Rustoen, 1995). Others (Tomko, 1985; Omer & Rosenbaum, 1997) caution that hope in some cases may compromise adjustment.

If hope is viewed as the perceived probability of goal attainment (Stotland, 1969), for patients faced with a serious illness and its associated losses, despair should well be expected. Spencer et al. (1997) suggest that the acknowledgement of despair over lost possibilities can actually lead to activation of the will to over-come. These authors note that experiencing illness-associated grief and despair is for many patients an important initial step in the process of hoping. Thus, honor-ing the process of grief work for patients around lost expectations and helping them realign objects of hope may in fact be essential for reality-based and endur-ing hopefulness. Moreover, hope, in particular unrealistic hope or exaggerated hope, comes at a price. It is well documented that decreased ability to predict the occurrence of an event is associated with greater distress (Henry & Wang, 1998). Thus, hope may interfere with anticipatory planning and preparation for bad news. Finally, as Tomko (1985) notes, hopefulness can be dysfunctional when its emotional expense outweighs its benefits.

HOPE AND DESPAIR: TWO SIDES OF THE COIN

Taken together, the literature describes various internal and external dimensions of the concept of hope. These dimensions vary significantly among individuals, deter-mined for the most part by personal values and goals. Particularly for those with medical illness, the inner experience of hope—finding personal meaning despite unfulfilled expectations—appears to be important to sustain an enduring hope. The existence of hope, however, does not preclude the experience of despair. Hope and despair can coexist, and some would argue, must coexist to be meaningful. Kegan's (1982) conceptualization of hope as "a dialectic between limits and possi-bilities" (p. 45) can be used to reconcile these divergent themes. It is important to consider hope's benefits as well as its costs. As Spencer et al. (1997) suggest, acknowledge the limits of hope, understand the associated emotions of despair and grief, and rejoice in the discovery of new future possibilities.

CLINICAL IMPLICATIONS

HOPE AS A PROCESS

Each patient brings his or her own blend of hope and reality to the illness situation, thus creating a uniquely personal view of the illness and of the future. Clinically, the challenge is to understand the patient's personal context and meaning of hopefulness. The intensity of the need for hope may depend on the patient's perceived threat to personal safety (Morse & Doberneck, 1995). Knowledge of the patient's needs and strengths can guide the balance between helping patients with reality testing and allowing them to create the essential illusions necessary to cope (Salander, Bergenheim, & Henriksson, 1996). Hope is a dynamic process that will likely change over time as the patient meets new challenges or obstacles. For hope to be enduring and adaptive, as much as possible for each individual, it should be rooted in reality. When hope is based on illusions fueled by false assurances, it can cause considerable anguish.

THE REALIGNMENT OF HOPE

Perhaps it is not so much a question of relinquishing hope, but rather of realigning objects of hope as events warrant. To illustrate, a patient upon learning of her disease recurrence explained hope realignment as follows:

> I keep rearranging the things in my life that I hope for. When I was getting chemo I hoped I wouldn't lose my hair. When I was finished my treatment my hope was to get my old life back as quick as possible. Now, I just hope to see my son graduate from high school next year. My cancer has taught me to hope for the best but prepare for the worst and trust in God's will.

Some specific intervention strategies (Morse & Doberneck, 1995) that can be useful in supporting reality-based hope include the following:

- A realistic assessment of threat
- The envisioning of alternatives and the setting of goals
- A bracing for negative outcomes
- A realistic assessment of personal resources and of external conditions and resources

- The solicitation of supportive relationships
- The continuous evaluation for signs that reinforce the selected goals or the need to modify the means to achieve the goal or the goal itself
- A determination to endure

It is important that patients, as much as possible, understand the medical reality, to have the opportunity to evaluate medical options and choices, and to plan for the future meaningfully. Other clinical implications include the following:

1. Assessing hope
2. Providing hope work interventions for patients and families
3. Tailoring medical communication to the needs of patients
4. Combining honesty with hopefulness
5. Providing ongoing support to both patients and families

ASSESSMENT OF HOPE

Regarding assessment, gather initial and subsequent hope assessments and related information guides as part of the clinical database. Some relevant questions are as follows: Are you hopeful or hopeless? What have been significant sources of hope for you in the past, currently, and for the future? What are your hopes for your recovery? What do you expect to be the outcome of your illness/your treatment? Who/what supports your hopefulness? Who/what threatens your hopefulness? What can you tell the oncology team about your information style preferences? How do you want to hear medical information: alone or with others present? Do you want detailed or more general information related to disease, treatment, and prognosis? Various instruments, for example the Herth Hope Scale (1992), can provide guidance when assessing hope for patients. If patients report being hopeless, a careful psychosocial assessment should follow, recognizing that hopelessness, in some, may be an indication of depression.

HOPE-ENHANCING STRATEGIES

Hope may be enhanced by various psychological interventions designed to provide meaning and increase one's sense of dignity and self-worth to face the future positively (Nunn, 1996). Listening to the patient's life story, appreciating what is personally meaningful to the patient, and understanding his or her lived experience of illness are helpful strategies to support hope. As Frankl (1984) noted, understanding one's purpose in life and the ability to make sense of one's experiences are often useful as means of sustaining hope. Specific hope-enhancing strategies also include prayer/religion, distraction (Raleigh, 1992), and coping behaviors, such as avoidance and positive reappraisal (Jarrett, Ramirez, Richards, & Weinman, 1992; Salander et al., 1996). The cognitive techniques of reframing, refocusing, and distraction may be particularly beneficial; that is, focusing on the positive aspects of situations and directing patients to stay present-centered and deal with problems as they arise, not as they are anticipated. Additionally, patients' spiritual needs and beliefs must be assessed and supported for their contribution to hopefulness.

FINDING HOPE THROUGH THE PRESENCE OF OTHERS

The importance of supportive, caring others in maintaining the hope of patients has been well documented (Post-White et al., 1996). However, some investigators have found that perceived future availability and adequacy of significant others may be actually more significant than current support (Nunn, 1996). As clinicians, it is important that we assess current as well as future adequacy of patients' support networks and mobilize those who will be central to the patient's care and well-being, raising their awareness of the importance of their physical and emotional availability to the patient.

SYMPTOM MANAGEMENT CAN SUPPORT HOPE

Promoting patient independence and control, as well as aggressive management of psychological and physical distress, will lessen helplessness and contribute to personal hopefulness. Behavioral techniques, such as stress management training, can enhance control, and supportive interventions may reduce isolation and increase a patient's connection with others, all contributing to personal hopefulness (Bunston et al., 1995; Nunn, 1996).

MINDFULNESS MEDITATION

A useful behavioral intervention is "mindfulness," a meditation strategy particularly useful to enhance hope. Mindfulness is a practice that can assist patients in refocusing hope from future to present orientation, because living in the moment can be an important source of hope. Borysenko (1994) describes mindfulness as a moment-by-moment, nonjudgmental awareness that can bring about a renewed sense of gratitude and peace. The practice of mindfulness is a useful strategy to bring a person to "present-centered awareness." Rinpoche (1994) describes present awareness as a way to bring the mind back home. Basically, to bring your mind home is to turn your mind inward and to rest in the nature of the mind without indulging in emotions or suppressing them. Instead, emotions and thoughts are viewed with an acceptance and generosity, while affirming the importance of the present moment: "The only thing I have is nowness, is now" (Rinpoche, 1994). This practice involves paying attention to whatever experience one might be having at the moment—fully experiencing "what is" with all the related sensations and feelings. For example, while eating savor the taste and texture of the food, or in the evening, marvel at the colors and majesty of a sunset. Mindfulness exercises can teach patients to place hope in the present by realizing the preciousness of the moment.

SUPPORTING PERSONAL HOPEFULNESS

There are many interventions to promote and sustain hope. Most important for clinical practice, understanding the hopes, beliefs, needs, and fears of each patient should serve as the guide for selecting appropriate individualized hope-enhancing strategies.

Because hope is a dynamic process, over time, patients and their loved ones may need guidance with negotiating and renegotiating changing goals and objectives.

We should anticipate that conflicts may arise when the need for truth versus hope differs for the patient and loved ones. Strain may take the form of family members blaming patients if their "hope" wavers and they lose their "fighting spirit." Patients may feel that family members are "living in a bubble" and "not accepting the reality of the illness." Above all, it is important to acknowledge and normalize the strain and support patients and family members to do the necessary grief work, proceed at their own pace when confronting painful realities associated with the disease, respect differences, and keep lines of communication open to resolve conflicts quickly.

OTHER UNFULFILLED HOPES

Pain and disappointment are expected when patients' hopes are not fulfilled and disease progresses; however, in some situations when hope is realized for remission or cure, there may still be disappointment because of other unfulfilled hopes and expectations. A patient completing treatment with an excellent prognosis illustrates this point:

> I expected all my family problems to vanish when treatment was over. I hoped the family learned, as I have come to learn, the preciousness of life and the stupidity of wasting energy bickering about trivial, inconsequential matters. But I was wrong and I am so disappointed. Not only are all the problems back, but I also feel completely alone now, because I no longer see these things as important and they do.

CLINICIANS' CONTRIBUTIONS TO HOPEFULNESS

Koopmeiners et al. (1997) explore specifically how health care professionals contribute to hope for patients with cancer. They have found that clinicians both positively and negatively influence hope. Hope is fostered by being present, demonstrating caring behaviors, giving information, and answering questions in a positive, honest, warm, polite, and respectful manner. Negative influences on hope include poor communication and conflicting information; physicians giving discouraging medical facts and information in a disrespectful, cold, or candid manner; and physicians trivializing the situation.

Similarly, Herth (1990) has found that devaluing human beings through degrading, belittling, patronizing comments, and noncaring responses threatens hope. Conversely, patients reported that having one's individuality respected fostered hope. Patients appreciate health care professionals treating them as worthwhile individuals despite their illness and declining physical function. Further, Nunn (1996) notes the perceived adequacy, reliability, and future availability of leadership figures, most important for patients with cancer, the physician and the oncology team, influence patients' hopefulness. Thus, we must assure the patient that he or she is valued, cared for, and will never be abandoned no matter what the medical outcome may be. It is imperative that clinicians not destroy patients' hopes with negative approaches that lack compassion.

COMMUNICATING BAD NEWS

Oncology clinicians, particularly physicians delivering bad news, face the daily challenge of how to balance truth telling with hope. Miyaji (1993) notes that the principle of hope as understood within the medical culture may conflict with the principle of truth telling. In a study of truth-telling practices among physicians, half of the physicians studied modified the information they provided if they believed the news would deprive their patients of hope. Moreover, bad news was often withheld, softened, or delayed to preserve the hope of patients, which as (Miyaji, 1993) noted was not objectively assessed and was subject to confounding with the physicians' own biases and needs. Further, most physicians believed that whether patients lost hope or not was their responsibility.

Similarly, Good, Good, Schaffer, and Lind (1990) have found that oncologists regulated the amount of information based on the desire to maintain their patients' hope. Thus, the importance of delivering bad news while still conveying a message of hope is well documented but not well researched (Ptacek & Eberhardt, 1996), well understood, or well implemented. From a synthesis of the literature, Ptacek and Eberhardt (1996) offer some specific physician recommendations: Deliver bad news in a private place, face to face in a supportive manner with a loved one present; explore what the patient or family want to know, and tailor the specificity of the news to the patient's needs; and allow patients to participate freely in the exchange of information. Hope should be truthfully conveyed; in the case of imminent death, hope may come from the physician's ability to control symptoms and minimize discomfort. Allow patients to express emotions, and help them work through their reactions. These recommendations are similar to patients' views of wanting to be told bad news in person, privately with a support person present. They wanted their physicians to be honest, compassionate, caring, hopeful, and informative (Peteet, Abrams, Ross, & Stearns, 1991). How medical news is delivered is just as important as what is actually said.

ACHIEVING A DELICATE BALANCE

Balancing information and hope with the patient's needs is an ongoing clinical challenge. As Nekolaichuk and Bruera (1998) note, false despair is equally as destructive as false hope. Full disclosure of medical information for some may not be desired or helpful, while for others, it may be absolutely essential. Providing truthful information while offering hope, which may range from promising treatments to end of life support, combined with knowing and respecting each patient can guide clinicians with this difficult task. Last, clinicians must be vigilant to avoid allowing personal beliefs and biases to interfere with the truthful, supportive, and timely delivery of medical information.

CLINICAL STRATEGIES

1. Comprehensively assess the patient's personal view of hope.
2. Use a variety of behavioral, psychological, and spiritual techniques tailored to the patient's needs to enhance hope.
3. Use meditation exercises, such as mindfulness, to shift awareness from future events to present moment; use various affirmations, such as "What is is and I can handle it" (Borysenko, 1994).
4. The development of specific objects of hope is an evolving process that allows patients to focus on concrete, realistic goals that are appropriate and attainable at any given point (eg, hope for the end of treatment, hope for full recovery, hope for a peaceful death).
5. Support patients and loved ones with necessary grief work related to lost hopes and expectations to build an enduring hope on reality, not on illusion.

6. Incorporate hope work into daily life. For example, realign and readjust objects of hope as necessary. Lower expectations, and find hope in small steps and gradual progress.
7. Be honest and supportive when delivering medical news, while respecting patient's preferences and needs.
8. The clinician's presence is, in itself, a significant source of hope.

CASE STUDY

A. L. was a 42-year-old divorced mother of two adolescents. She was initially diagnosed with metastatic breast cancer approximately 3 years ago. At the time of diagnosis, A. L. sought a second opinion from an expert medical oncologist. During this consultation visit, A. L. was told that she had a very aggressive disease, and she had no more than 3 years to live. This interaction devastated her. As A. L. reported, "the doctor bludgeoned me with this medical news. I have lived with a death sentence hanging over my head for almost 3 years." At the approach of the third year, A. L developed a significant clinical depression. She was hopeless, suicidal, and believed she would not live beyond the year, even though her disease was well controlled at the time. As A. L. stated, "that doctor was the expert. If he told me I would be dead, he must be right."

Clinicians must appreciate the powerful impact of their words and manner on patients. As patients are faced with the diagnosis of cancer, they are often in a vulnerable state. At the very least, professionals must choose their words thoughtfully and communicate supportively, to avoid destroying hope and adding to the burden of this disease. What may simply be viewed as a casual comment to a patient, quickly forgotten by the clinician, may become an albatross for the patient for a long time to come.

REFERENCES

Ballard, A., Green, T., McCaa, A., & Logsdon, C. M. (1997). A comparison of the level of hope in patients with newly diagnosed and recurrent cancer. *Oncology Nursing Forum, 24*(5), 899–904.

Bennett, M. I., & Bennett, M. B. (1984). The uses of hopelessness. *American Journal of Psychiatry, 141,* 559–562.

Dufault, K., & Martocchio, B. C. (1985). Hope: Its spheres and dimensions. *Nursing Clinics of North America, 20*(2), 379–391.

Borysenko, J. (1994). *Pocketful of miracles.* New York: Warner Books.

Beck, A. T., Steer, R. A., Kovacs, M., & Garrison, G. (1985). Hopelessness and eventual suicide: A 10 year prospective study of patients. *American Journal of Psychiatry, 142,* 559–563.

Brockopp, D. Y., Hayko, D., Davenport, W., & Winscott, C. (1989). Personal control and the needs for hope and information among adults diagnosed with cancer. *Cancer Nursing, 12,* 112–116.

Bunston, T., Mings, D., Mackie, A., & Jones, D. (1995). Facilitating hopefulness: The determinants of hope. *Journal of Psychosocial Oncology, 13*(4), 79–99.

Christman, N. J. (1990). Uncertainty and adjustment during radiotherapy. *Nursing Research, 39,* 17–20.

Ellison, C. W. (1983). Spiritual well-being: Conceptualization and measurement. *Journal of Psychology and Theology, 11,* 330–340.

Ersek, M. (1992). The process of maintaining hope in adults undergoing bone marrow transplantation for leukemia. *Oncology Nursing Forum, 19,* 883–889.

Frankl, V. (1984). Man's search for meaning. New York: Washington Square Press.

Good, M. D., Good, B. J., Schaffer, C., & Lind, S. E., (1990). American oncology and the discourse on hope. *Cultural Medical Psychiatry, 14*(1), 59–79.

Greer, S. (1992). The management of denial in cancer patients. *Oncology, 6*(12), 33–40.

Henry, J. P., & Wang, S. (1998). Effects of early stress on adult affiliative behavior. *Psychoneuroendocrinology, 23,* 863–875.

Herth, K. (1990). Fostering hope in terminally ill people. *Journal of Advanced Nursing, 18,* 538–548.

Herth, K. (1991). Development and refinement of an instrument to measure hope. *Scholarly Inquiry for Nursing Practice: An International Journal, 5* (1), 39–51.

Herth, K. (1992). Abbreviated instrument to measure hope: Development and psychometric evaluation. *Journal of Advanced Nursing, 17,* 1251–1259.

Hinds, P. S. (1984). Inducing a definition of "hope" through the use of grounded theory methodology. *Journal of Advanced Nursing, 18,* 538–548.

Hinds, P. S. & Martin, J. (1988). Hopefulness and the self-sustaining process in adolescents with cancer. *Nursing Research, 37*(6), 336–340.

Jarrett, S. R., Ramirez, A. J., Richards, M. A., & Weinman, J. (1992). Measuring coping in breast cancer. *Journal of Psychosomatic Research,* 593.

Kegan, R. (1982). *The evolving self: Problems and process in human development.* Cambridge, MA: Harvard University Press.

Koopmeiners, L., Post-White, J., Gutknecht, S., Ceronsky, C., Nickelson, K., Drew, D., Mackey, K. W., & Kreitzer, M. J. (1997). How healthcare professionals contribute to hope in patients with cancer. *Oncology Nursing Forum, 24*(9), 1507–1513.

Kubler-Ross, E. (1969). *On death and dying.* New York: Macmillan.

Lazarus, R. S., & Folkman, S. (1984). Stress appraisal and coping. New York: Springer.

Mahon, S. M., Cella, D. F., & Donovan, M. I. (1990). Psychosocial adjustment to recurrent cancer. *Oncology Nursing Forum, 17,* 7–52.

Miyaji, N. T. (1993). The power of compassion: Truth-telling among American doctors in the care of dying patients. *Social Science Medicine, 36*(3), 249–264.

Morse, J. M., & Doberneck, B. (1995). Delineating the concept of hope. *Image: Journal of Nursing Scholarship, 27,* 277–285.

Nekolaichuk, C. L., & Bruera, E. (1998). On the nature of hope in palliative care. *Journal of Palliative Care, 14*(1), 36–42.

Nunn, K. P. (1996). Personal hopefulness: A conceptual review of the relevance of the perceived future to psychiatry. *British Journal of Medical Psychology, 69,* 227–245.

Omer, H., & Rosenbaum, R. (1997). Diseases of hope and the work of despair. *Psychotherapy, 34*(3), 225–232.

Pascal. 1984. Thoughts, 47. In Comte-Sponville, *Traite du desespoir et de la beatitude.* Paris: Presses Universitaires de France.

Peteet, J., Abrams, H., Ross, D. M., & Stearns, N. M. (1991). Presenting a diagnosis of cancer: Patients' views. *Journal Family Practice, 2,* 577–581.

Post-White, J., Ceronsky, C., Kreitzer, M. J., Nickelson, K., Drew, D., Mackey, K. W., Koopmeiners, L., & Gutknecht, S. (1996). Hope, spirituality, sense of coherence, and quality of life in patients with cancer. *Oncology Nursing Forum, 23*(10), 1571–1579.

Proverbs 13:12.

Ptacek, J. T., & Eberhardt, T. L. (1996). Breaking bad news. *Journal of the American Medical Association, August 14, 276*(6), 496–502.

Raleigh, E. D., (1992). Sources of hope in chronic illness. *Oncology Nursing Forum, 19,* 443–447.

Rinpoche, S. (1993). The Tibetan handbook of living and dying. San Francisco: Harper.

Rustoen, T. (1995). Hope and quality of life. *Cancer Nursing, 18*(5), 355–361.

Salander, P., Bergenheim, T., Henriksson, R. (1996). The creation of protection and hope in patients with malignant brain tumours. *Social Science Medicine, 42*(7), 985–996.

Spencer, J., Davidson, H., & White, V. (1997). Helping clients develop hopes for the future. *The American Journal of Occupational Therapy, 51*(3), 191–198.

Spinoza. *Ethics, Part III, explication of definition 13.*

Stoner, M. H. (1983). Hope and cancer patients. *Dissertation Abstracts International, 44*(1-B).

Stotland, E. (1969). *The psychology of hope.* San Francisco: Jossey-Bass.

Tomko, B. (1985). The burden of hope. *Hospice Journal, 1*(3), 91–97.

Weiner, B. (1985). An attribution theory of achievement motivation and emotion. *Psychological Review, 92,* 548–573.

Waiting symbolizes to me that hope never dies.

I was diagnosed with breast cancer in July
1998. A mastectomy and chemotherapy
followed. When the chemo was finished,
I checked every morning for signs that my
hair was coming back—a new beginning.

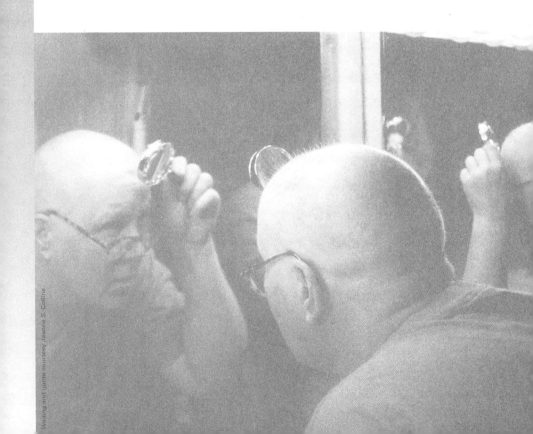

CHAPTER 4

Uncertainty

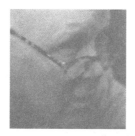

"Anyone looking honestly at life will see that we live in a constant state of suspense and ambiguity. Our minds are perpetually shifting in and out of confusion and clarity. . . . What is really baffling about life is that sometimes, despite all our confusion, we can also be really wise!" (Rinpoche, 1994, pp. 104–105)

DISCUSSION OF THE LITERATURE

When a chronic illness intrudes, it sharply separates the person of the present from the person of the past and affects or even shatters any images of the self held for the future (Corbin & Strauss, 1988). Cancer, with its often insidious, ambiguous presentation and unpredictable course, takes the experience of uncertainty to a higher level. As Mages and Mendelsohn (1982) note, cancer can be a continuing, unremitting condition of uncertainty about potentially disastrous and poorly predictable future events.

ILLNESS-RELATED UNCERTAINTY

Illness-related uncertainty has been defined as the inability to determine the meaning of illness events when these events are ambiguous, highly complex, lacking information, or when outcomes cannot be predicted (Mishel, 1988; 1990). As a construct, uncertainty has both perceptive and cognitive components (Mishel, 1981). Hilton (1988) notes that uncertainty is a perceptual state that exists on a continuum and changes over time. The uncertainty of living with chronic illness has been the subject of study in various disciplines, particularly in nursing. Since Mishel's (1981) early work, there has been significant scientific study of the construct of uncertainty. For an excellent review on this topic, see Mast's (1995) critical review of the adult uncertainty research.

Mishel (1988; 1990) developed a theoretical model of uncertainty in illness organized around four categories:

1. Antecedent factors, which precede and contribute to the perception of uncertainty, such as illness severity, personal beliefs, and social support
2. Uncertainty and its personal appraisal as threat or opportunity
3. Problem-focused and emotion-focused coping
4. Adaptation

Outcomes research examining uncertainty in illness has shown an association between uncertainty and adjustment (Oberst & Scott, 1985), distress (Wineman, Schwetz, Goodkin, & Rudick, 1996; Wong & Bramwell, 1992), spiritual well-being (Landis, 1996), coping (Christman et al., 1988; Mishel, 1988), and quality of life (Hawthorne & Hixon, 1994).

PERSONAL PERCEPTION OF UNCERTAINTY

While uncertainty in chronic illness is likely to differ across the experience of illness (Mishel, 1996) and take on varying degrees of significance in different illnesses (Wiener & Dodd, 1993), the personal perception of uncertainty appears to play a major role in uncertainty appraisal and coping. An illness, to be understood, must be placed in a biographical context—what was going on before, what life was like in the past, what hopes and dreams were interrupted or changed (Corbin & Strauss, 1988). Thus, it is important to understand the individual's experience of illness-related uncertainty within its highly personal life context. Uncertainty in cancer is uniquely experienced by each individual depending on his or her interpretation of cancer (for example, punishment, curse, embarrassment; Sontag, 1978), tolerance for uncertainty, degree of disruption from the illness, social support, and personal need for control (Wiener & Dodd, 1993). However, there does not appear to be a consistent relationship between illness severity, progression, and uncertainty. As Mast (1995) noted, it's unlikely that illness characteristics alone are adequate predictors of uncertainty. Rather, an individual's perception of uncertainty arises from the interaction of illness-related situational factors as well as personal factors (Hilton, 1988; 1989).

As Mishel (1995) notes, uncertainty appraisal is mediated by inference and illusion. Because the characteristics of an uncertain situation are that it is unclear, vague, and unpredictable, patients often form a personal belief system to redefine the situation into one that is understandable and controllable (Mishel, 1993; 1996). Patients need to construct personal meaning of the illness to understand the event within their own lived experience and to manage the associated distress.

Further, Wineman, Durand, and Steiner (1994) emphasize the importance of personal vulnerability as an antecedent variable to uncertainty. The appraisal of a situation as dangerous and the perception of a high level of uncertainty, hence vulnerability, results in a greater disturbance in emotional well-being (Wineman et al.).

DANGER VERSUS OPPORTUNITY

Whether an individual appraises illness-related uncertainty as a danger or as an opportunity appears to influence significantly emotional response and coping. As Mishel (1995) notes, coping strategies may mediate between uncertainty, appraisal, and psychosocial adaptation. It appears, for the most part, when uncertainty is appraised as a danger, there is increased emotional arousal, and emotion-focused coping strategies (such as escape–avoidance) are often used to regulate the distress. When uncertainty is perceived as an opportunity, problem-focused behaviors (such as information-seeking) are used to alter the situation; however, some individuals may use both problem-focused and emotion-focused coping following a danger appraisal (Mishel, 1995).

When uncertainty is viewed as a danger, the uncertainty itself may create further distress, which in turn has an adverse effect on coping and adjustment (Landis, 1996; Lazarus & Folkman, 1984). With persistent uncertainty, coping resources may become ineffective and further reduce the amount of adaptive energy available for mobilizing resources. Depletion of adaptive energy may move individuals into an impoverished adaptive state, placing them at risk for further impairments (Landis, 1996).

COPING STRATEGIES

It is unclear which coping strategies or combination of coping strategies may effectively reduce the emotional distress associated with uncertainty (Mast, 1995). Investigators have found that the specific coping strategies used had little impact on the effect of uncertainty on emotional distress (Wineman et al., 1994; Mishel & Sorenson, 1991). Moreover, individuals who report moderate to severe psychological distress are more likely to experience illness uncertainty (Mast, 1998; Wong & Bramwell, 1992). Perhaps the level of psychological distress influences the perception of uncertainty, particularly when the degree of uncertainty is not congruent with medical events.

> I feel like I am on a raft with a slow leak in the middle of the ocean. Even though I've been told by all my doctors that my prognosis is excellent and I can expect full and complete recovery, I feel that my fate is sealed. Cancer is so unpredictable that I can't be certain of anything. I can't even be certain that I will see tomorrow.

On the other hand, uncertainty may provide opportunities for insight and personal growth (Mishel, 1988; 1990) through reevaluation of life values, goals, and priorities (Belec, 1992; Cella & Tross, 1986). With chronic illness, individuals may abandon the search for predictability and certainty and gradually come to view uncertainty not only as inevitable, but also as an opportunity for positive change. As Rinpoche (1994) notes, the uncertainty of life "creates gaps, spaces in which profound changes and opportunities for transformation are continuously flowering—if, that is, they can be seen and seized" (p. 105).

> I am so grateful for my illness. It has taught me how important life is. I am so much more appreciative for each day because I'm not sure how many more days I will have. But for the extra time I have been given—I really live my life and I don't waste it on unimportant worries and foolish concerns.

AN UNCERTAIN WORLD

Once you become a "cancer patient," you must learn to live in an uncertain world. Across the cancer trajectory, individuals will likely experience increased uncertainty at various crisis or transition points over the course of their illness. As Mishel (1996) notes, coping with uncertainty in chronic illness is a complex process and likely to change over time as the nature and source of the uncertainty change. While the amount of uncertainty perceived by individuals with similar types of cancer varies (Christman, 1990), there are discernible patterns to consider.

PATTERNS OF UNCERTAINTY

One perspective to view the uncertainty of cancer is Mishel's (1993) categorization of symptom uncertainty, medical uncertainty, and daily living uncertainty (Mishel, 1993). Symptom uncertainty refers to difficulties distinguishing a pattern to the symptoms. Medical uncertainty involves difficulty with diagnosis, treatment options, side effects, and sorting out their effects and management. Daily living uncertainty includes the impact of the person's illness and treatment on activities of daily living. After treatment ends, uncertainty about recurrence may cause patients to be vigilant and monitor themselves closely, often with difficulty in distinguishing the normal from abnormal (Mishel, 1993; 1996).

Additionally, Cohen (1993) added etiologic uncertainty as common in people with cancer who have followed a healthy lifestyle and have no explanation for the occurrence of the malignancy. When patients are uncertain as to the cause of cancer, they will construct personal explanations. These explanations are subjectively formed and may not have a basis in medical science (Mishel, 1996). Personal explanations may include attributional strategies to assign responsibility, such as self-blame, other-blame, punishment for wrongdoing, and so on (Hilton, 1989). As Folkman (1984) notes, the more ambiguous a situation is, the more inference is required and the more personal factors will influence the appraisal. Fear may produce the need for convincing reassurances gained through mechanisms such as selective inattention and recall (Janis, 1967). Thus, there is an interaction, a negotiation between expectations and what is really happening (Gevins et al., 1987). In essence, patients fill in the gaps to create meaning and enhance control in ambiguous, threatening situations. These personal interpretations can include bits of medical facts coupled with pieces of personal conjecture.

A patient with metastatic breast cancer who had failed three treatments met with her doctor who realistically laid out the limited treatment options in a clear but gentle manner. After the meeting, the patient told her nurse, "The doctor told me that we do have fewer options now than before, but not to worry, there are still a million treatments that we can try."

AN UNCERTAIN BODY

Wiener and Dodd (1993) offer another perspective to view the uncertainty of cancer within the context of three interrelated elements: temporality, body, and identity. Loss of temporal predictability, duration, and frequency can be illustrated by statements such as, "How long will this illness last?" or "When is my treatment going to end?" The body element consists of disruptions related to the uncertain body and body failure; for example, the body's inability to perform an activity, appearance, physiological functioning, and response to treatment illustrate the patient's shaken faith in the "taken-for-granted body." Last, uncertain identity is an important element. "Do I really have cancer? I feel fine." Shifts in identity may necessitate giving up past conceptions of self. "Who am I now? I don't recognize myself." In response to these troubling elements of uncertainty, individuals strive to gain control of the situation.

As a patient beginning chemotherapy expressed, "I have constant images of the cancer eating away at my insides. I just can't get these thoughts out of my head. It's like the cancer has taken over my body, my mind, and my life." Another patient facing bone marrow transplantation noted, "All I want is my old life back."

UNCERTAINTY AND SOCIAL SUPPORT

In terms of uncertainty and social support, the data suggest that supportive relationships may assist individuals to make cognitive sense of the illness experience with generally a corresponding lessening in the distress related to uncertainty (Mast, 1995). Further, there has been some study of uncertainty in family members and of differing perceptions of uncertainty in various ethnic groups. For example, Northouse, Laten, and Reddy (1995) found that women with recurrent breast cancer and their husbands differed in reported uncertainty, with spouses reporting more uncertainty than patients did. Germino et al. (1998) studied patient and family patterns of coping with uncertainty related to prostate cancer among white and African American families. They found differences and similarities between patients and family members and between ethnic groups. For all, however, uncertainty was associated with psychological distress. Finally, limited outcome studies have examined the efficacy of strategies to manage illness-related uncertainty. In a recent work, Braden, Mishel, and Longman (1998) studied self-care promotion and uncertainty management interventions for women receiving breast cancer treatment. These interventions resulted in higher levels of self-care, self-help, psychological adjustment, and confidence in cancer knowledge.

COMPLEXITY OF UNCERTAINTY

Taken together, uncertainty is a pervasive feature of chronic illness. There is a complex interaction of personal and situational factors in the appraisal of uncertainty. Uncertainty has been consistently associated with emotional distress, reduced quality of life, and compromised psychosocial adjustment. However, there is evidence that uncertainty may provide benefit to some when viewed as an opportunity rather than as a danger. In general, individuals use a combination of emotion-focused and problem-focused techniques to cope with uncertainty. The particular coping strategies used, however, seem to have little impact on distress reduction. There has been little comparative study of the experience of uncertainty for family members and for various ethnic groups and limited study of the efficacy of uncertainty interventions. However, several clinical implications can be derived from this rich body of literature to guide practice.

CLINICAL IMPLICATIONS

Central to clinical management is the clinician's understanding of the patient's experience of uncertainty. Clinicians should view uncertainty within the larger context of the patient's life experiences, medical situation, and psychological response.

ASSESSMENT OF UNCERTAINTY

Patients need comprehensive assessment at regular intervals, particularly during points of transition. Assess psychological status, concurrent stressors, coping skills, and available supports. Do a narrative assessment of the patient's fears, hopes, areas of vulnerability, and strengths. How vulnerable does the patient feel? Ascertain if patients view illness-related uncertainty as a danger or opportunity for growth. Patients who perceive uncertainty as a danger may be at greater risk for emotional distress (Mishel et al., 1991). Exaggerated uncertainty out of proportion to the medical situation or high levels interfering with functioning may suggest psychological disturbances, such as post-traumatic stress disorder (PTSD), anxiety, or depressive disorders with the associated vulnerability and perceptions of uncontrollability and danger. Perform a comprehensive psychological assessment.

Additionally, symptom distress, concurrent illness problems, and fear of recurrence may contribute to perceptions of uncertainty (Mast, 1998). Complete a physical assessment to assess pain, fatigue, nausea, sleep problems, and so on, all of which potentially contribute to the uncontrollability and uncertainty of the medical situation. Help patients develop a plan with reasonable expectations of control.

Anticipate that crisis points can be triggers for increased anxiety and uncertainty. Closely assess uncertainty levels during these times.

INDIVIDUALIZED PLAN OF SUPPORT

Assess the patient's usual coping style, tolerance for uncertainty, and level of distress to put in place coping strategies that are individually tailored. These strategies may include problem-focused coping, such as information seeking, problem-solving strategies, mobilizing social support, or emotion-focused strategies, which include positive reframing, minimization, and emotional distancing. Assess the patient's spiritual needs and well-being, and identify meaningful areas of support.

Uncertainty may be exacerbated if individuals are unable to discern a consistent pattern in their symptoms, if illness-related information is not provided or not understood (Mishel, 1988), and if patients fail to anticipate illness symptoms and events (Mast, 1995). Moreover, inadequate information from health professionals and ambiguity regarding future procedures can create further uncertainty for patients (Loveys & Klaich, 1991; Weems & Patterson, 1989; Weiner & Dodd, 1993), while trust and confidence in the health care providers may significantly reduce uncertainty (Mishel & Braden, 1988). Thus, it is important to provide clear, understandable information regarding expected side effects of medications and treatments to assist patients to sort out the meaning of various physical and psychological changes.

- Explain what is likely to occur as side effects of treatment, as opposed to signs of disease progression.
- Explain planned procedures, and warn patients of anticipated medical events.
- Teach self-care skills.
- Answer patients' questions thoroughly, and provide ongoing information as indicated.
- Assist patients to develop personally meaningful interpretations of illness.
- Support patients as they grieve over lost certainties, such as health and independence, and reformulate personal identity over the course of the illness.
- Assist patients with reordering of life priorities and goals.
- Maximize the growth-producing potential of uncertainty.

Uncertainty and fear may produce a strong need for vigilant behavior, manifested by increased attentiveness and readiness to take protective action (Janis, 1967); this is heightened when individuals perceive that protection is primarily dependent on their individual actions (Reutter & Northcott, 1994). It is thus important for patients to understand that they are not alone in the management of their illness. We are the patients' advocates, and we need to understand the importance of this role to help patients feel safe.

On the other hand, clinicians must recognize that some patients may actually prefer uncertainty to certainty, especially in situations where options are limited or prognosis is bleak. As a patient explained, "I don't want to hear the statistics and prognosis. It's better for me not to know rather than hear the worst." Patients' information needs must be assessed and respected.

LIVING WITH UNCERTAINTY

Uncertainty doesn't end when treatment is completed. For cancer survivors, research suggests that the potential for illness uncertainty is a significant continuing stressor (Maher, 1982; Mast, 1998) and may strongly influence a person's adaptive behavior (Mast, 1998). In addition, the fear of cancer returning and distressing physical symptoms may contribute directly to emotional distress (Mast, 1998). Cancer patients who are able to view cancer, in some measure, as positive and growth producing may be better able to balance the uncertainty, the emotional strain, and the physical discomfort that may accompany cancer survival (Mishel, 1990; Moch, 1989; Mast, 1998).

UNCERTAINTY ABATEMENT WORK

Wiener and Dodd (1993) describe "uncertainty abatement work" as a combination of various activities to reduce the impact of the uncertainty of time, body, and identity. These activities include the following:

- Pacing, modifying, and reworking a schedule of daily activities

- Becoming professional patients, learning as much as possible about management of the disease
- Seeking reinforcing comparisons: downward comparisons ("this could be much worse") and upward comparisons ("others have survived a similar illness")
- Engaging in reviews; creating personal meaning of the experience of illness
- Setting goals; identifying short-term goals as focal points for certainty
- Covering up; hiding feelings so that *cancer patient* is not one's primary public identity
- Finding a safe place to let down, to share distress with those who are able to understand and support
- Choosing a supportive network; selectively sharing illness information with those who are likely to offer support rather than create more distress
- Taking charge; making decisions about the illness and its management

MANAGING UNCERTAINTY

Additionally, Mishel (1995; 1996) identifies strategies for managing illness uncertainty depending on the focus of the uncertainty, for example, for etiologic and symptom uncertainty, forming illness schema, constructing a normative framework, and using benchmarks. This includes providing a personal explanation for the illness, its causes, and its course and identifying self-care behaviors, for example, exercise programs, dietary modifications, support groups, and mind–body techniques. This assists patients to exercise control and mastery over their lives. Formulating timetables, such as a date when hair will return after chemotherapy, and benchmarks, such as improved energy levels, or reduced pain, to indicate progress.

For daily living uncertainty, Mishel (1995) identifies specifying controllable circumstances, using ritualistic behavior, and incorporating uncertainty into daily life. This includes controlling events; managing pain, sleep problems, and fatigue to minimize impact on daily routines; using behavioral reduction of uncertainty, such as exercising and practicing meditation; and changing attitudes to lessen the impact of uncertainty, for example lowering expectations of personal control and predictability in daily life.

At crisis or transition points, such as diagnosis, end of treatment, and recurrence, help patients anticipate and manage heightened uncertainty and mobilize emotional support.

- Advise patients to expect uncertainty and prepare for it. Support effective coping strategies, and encourage patients' reliance on their inner strength and personal resources.
- Assess stressful life events, both past and present, that may be contributing to the level of uncertainty.
- Keep life as predictable and normal as possible.
- Reduce as much as possible concurrent stressors.
- Provide aggressive symptom management, ongoing teaching, clear communication, and support.
- Rituals gain importance in proportion to the degree of uncertainty experienced (Roth, 1957). Assist patients to put in place meaningful activities that provide hope and relief, such as attending support groups, meditation, prayer.
- Create an environment of safety, clarity, and support to minimize the ambiguity and unpredictability related to the illness.
- Assess the experience of uncertainty for loved ones (may be a different course and experience).
- Address the role-related changes and associated uncertainty for patients, family members, and impact on family functioning.
- Provide information, support, and guidance to distinguish between anticipated and actual problems.

CLINICAL STRATEGIES

1. During and after treatment, assess for illness uncertainty and its associated distress.
2. Assessments should seek information about personal view of uncertainty (danger or opportunity), meaning of illness, tolerance for uncertainty, loss of control, coping style, concurrent stressors, symptom distress, fears about cancer recurrence, impact on family, and sources of support.
3. Through education and counseling, provide anticipatory guidance and assistance with known sources of illness uncertainty during and following completion of treatment.
4. Help patients work through their fears of disease recurrence and uncertainty, and assist in the exploration of potential growth-producing aspects of the cancer experience.
5. Assess and support loved ones as they cope with the illness-related uncertainty relevant to relationship and role changes.

CASE STUDY

PM was a 35-year-old patient newly diagnosed with melanoma. She presented with high levels of uncertainty and distress shortly after learning of her diagnosis. She noted the following:

All the terrifying experiences that I have been through in my life now come back to haunt me. I not only have to deal with the present uncertainty of the cancer and treatment, but also with my past uncertainties of what would happen to me after my parents' divorce when I was 7, after my mother's illness when I was 13. And, on top of all of this, I find myself constantly worrying about all the future uncertainties about my family. What if my daughter gets sick? What if my son gets hit by a car while riding his bike? What if my husband loses his job? I am so vulnerable and out of control. Life is no longer certain. There are no rules to follow, anything can happen. I have no protection.

I feel like I'm walking on thin ice with cracks all around. One misstep and everything comes crashing down. I'll feel a little better after my doctor tells me of my early stage and good prognosis and then something minor might happen and I'm once again devastated. The comfort of certainty is so fragile and can be easily shattered.

PM was referred for psychiatric evaluation and diagnosed with PTSD. Treatment included antidepressant therapy and counseling to which she responded over time. Specifically during counseling, the uncertainty management techniques used focused on positive reappraisal, viewing the cancer event as a challenge rather than a danger. This created an opportunity for PM to mobilize her considerable coping skills that served her well during her prior life crises. Guidance was also provided to PM to examine her lifestyle to identify and reduce controllable stressors. Through prioritizing her values and goals, PM reduced her work schedule to have more time to spend with her children. Through these and other techniques, PM was gradually able to reduce distress, regain personal confidence, and exercise control over her illness situation.

REFERENCES

Belec, R. H. (1992). Quality of life perceptions of long-term survivors of bone marrow transplantation. *Oncology Nursing Forum, 19*(1), 31–37.

Braden, C. J., Mishel, M. H., & Longman, A. J. (1998). Self help intervention project. Women receiving breast cancer treatment. *Cancer Practice, 6*(2), 87–98.

Cella, D. F., & Tross, S. (1986). Psychological adjustment to survival from Hodgkin's disease. *Journal of Consulting and Clinical Psychology, 54,* 616–622.

Christman, N. J. (1990). Uncertainty and adjustment during radiotherapy. *Nursing Research, 39*(1), 17–20.

Christman, N. J., McConnell, E. A., Pfeiffer, C., Webster, K. K., Schmitt, M., & Ries, J. (1988). Uncertainty, coping and distress following myocardial infarction: transition from hospital to home. *Research in Nursing & Health, 11,* 71–82.

Cohen, M. H. (1993). The unknown and the unknowable—Managing sustained uncertainty. *Western Journal of Nursing Research, 15,* 77–96.

Corbin, J., & Strauss, A. (1988). *Unending work and care.* San Francisco: Jossey Bass.

Folkman, S. (1984). Personal control and stress and coping processes: A theoretical analysis. *Journal of Personality and Social Psychology, 46*(4), 839–852.

Gevins, A., Morgan, N., Bressler, S., Cutello, B., White, R., Illes, J., Greer, D., Doyle, J., & Zeitlin, G. (1987). Human neuroelectric patterns predict performance accuracy. *Science, 235,* 550–585.

Germino, B. B., Mishel, M. H., Belyea, M., Harris, L., Ware, A., & Mohler, J. (1998). Uncertainty in prostate cancer. Ethnic and family patterns. *Cancer Practice, 6*(2), 107–113.

Hawthorne, M. H., & Hixon, M. E. (1994). Functional status, mood disturbance, and quality of life in patients with heart failure. *Progress in Cardiovascular Nursing, 9,* 22–32.

Hilton, B. A. (1988). The phenomenon of uncertainty in women with breast cancer. *Issues in Mental Health nursing, 9,* 217–238.

Hilton, B. A. (1989). The relationship of uncertainty, control, commitment, and threat of recurrence to coping strategies used by women diagnosed with breast cancer. *Journal of Behavioral Medicine, 12*(1), 39–54.

Janis, I. L. (1967). Effects of fear arousal on attitude change. Recent developments in theory and experimental research. In L. Berkowitz (Ed.), *Advances in experimental social psychology* (pp. 166–224.) New York: Academic Press.

Landis, B. J. (1996). Uncertainty, spiritual well-being, and psychosocial adjustment to chronic illness. *Issues in Mental Health Nursing, 17*(3), 217–231.

Lazarus, R. S., & Folkman, S. (1984). *Stress, appraisal, and coping.* New York: Springer.

Loveys, B. J., & Klaich, K. (1991). Breast cancer: Demands of illness. *Oncology Nursing Forum.*

Mages, N. L., & Mendelsohn, G. A. (1982). *Effects of cancer on patients' lives: A personological approach. Health Psychology: A Handbook* (pp. 252–284). San Francisco: Jossey Bass.

Maher, E. (1982). Anomic aspects of recovery from cancer. *Social Science and Medicine, 16,* 907–912.

Mast. M. E. (1995). Adult uncertainty in illness: A critical review of research. *Scholarly Inquiry for Nursing Practice, 9*(1), 3–29.

Mast, M. E. (1998). Survivors of breast cancer: Illness uncertainty, positive reappraisal and emotional distress. *Oncology Nursing Forum, 25*(3), 555–562.

Mishel, M. H. (1981). The measurement of uncertainty in illness. *Nursing Research, 30,* 258–263.

Mishel, M. H. (1988). Uncertainty in illness. *Image: Journal of Nursing Scholarship, 20,* 225–232.

Mishel, M. H. (1990). Reconceptualization of the uncertainty in illness theory. *Image: Journal of Nursing Scholarship, 22,* 256–262.

Mishel, M. H. (1993). Living with chronic illness: Living with uncertainty. In S. G. Funk, E. M. Tornquist, M. T. Champagne, & R. A. Wiese (Eds.), *Key aspects of caring for the chronically ill* (p. 46–58). New York: Springer.

Mishel, M. H. (1996). Commentary to: Uncertainty and coping in fathers of children with cancer. *Journal of Pediatric Nurses, 13*(2), 89–90.

Mishel, M. H., & Braden, C. J. (1988). Finding meaning: Antecedents of uncertainty in illness. *Nursing Research, 37,* 98–103.

Mishel, M. H., Padilla, G., Grant, M., & Sorenson, D. S. (1991). Uncertainty in illness theory: A replication of the mediating effects of mastery and coping. *Nursing Research, 40,* 236–240.

Mishel, M. H., & Sorenson, D. S. (1991). Uncertainty in gynecological cancer: A test of the mediating functions of mastery and coping. *Nursing Research, 40,* 167–171.

Moch, S. D. (1989). Health within illness: Conceptual evolution and practice possibilities. *Advances in Nursing Science, 11*(4), 23–31.

Northouse, L. L., Laten, D., & Reddy, P. (1995). Adjustment of women and their husbands to recurrent breast cancer. *Research in Nursing & Health, 18,* 515–524.

Oberst, M. T., Scott, D. (1985). Going home: Patient and spouse adjustment following cancer surgery. *Topics in Clinical Nursing, 7*(1), 46–57.

Reutter, L. I., & Northcott, H. C. (1994). Achieving a sense of control in a context of uncertainty: Nurses and AIDS. *Qualitative Health Research, 4*(1), 51–71.

Rinpoche, S. (1994). *The Tibetan book of living and dying.* San Francisco: Harper.

Roth, J. (1957). Ritual and magic in the control of contagion. *American Sociological Review, 22,* 310–314.

Sontag, S. (1978). *Illness as a metaphor.* New York: Farrar, Straus, & Giroux.

Sterken, D. J. (1996). Uncertainty and coping in fathers of children with cancer. *Journal of Pediatric Oncology Nurses, 13*(2), 81–88.

Weems, J., & Patterson, E. T. (1989). Coping with uncertainty and ambivalence while awaiting a cadaveric renal transplant. *Anna Journal, 16,* 27–31.

Wiener, C. L., & Dodd, M. J. (1993). Coping amid uncertainty: an illness trajectory perspective. *Scholarly Inquiry for Nursing Practice: An International Journal, 7*(1), 17–31.

Wineman, N. M., Durand, E. J., & Steiner, R. P. (1994). A comparative analysis of coping behaviors in persons with multiple sclerosis or a spinal cord injury. *Research in Nursing and Health, 17,* 185–194.

Wineman, N. M., Schwetz, K. M., Goodkin, D. E., & Rudick, R. A. (1996). Relationships among illness uncertainty, stress, coping, and emotional well-being at entry into a drug trial. *Applied Nursing Research, 9*(2), 53–60.

Wong, C., & Bramwell, L. (1992). Uncertainty and anxiety after mastectomy for breast cancer. *Issues in Mental Health Nursing, 15,* 363–371.

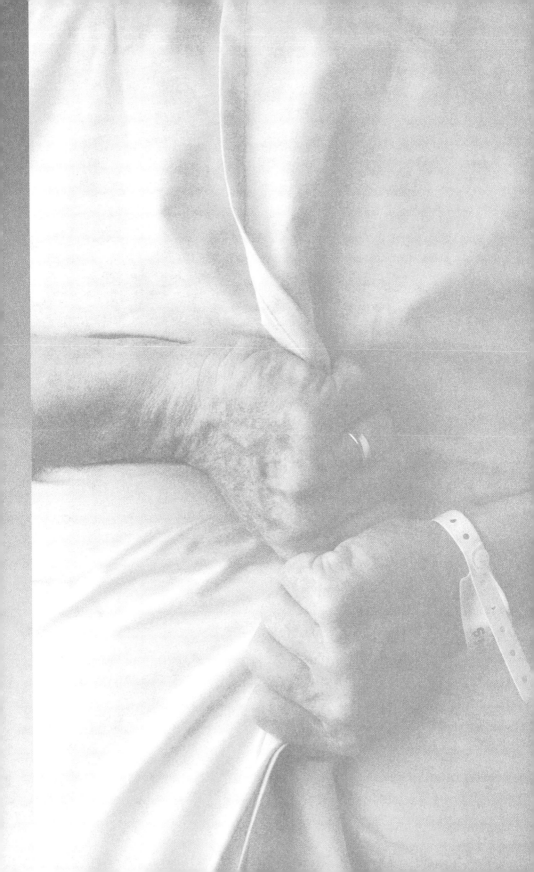

CHAPTER 5

Control

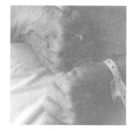

*"The fidelity of our
bodies is so basic that we
never think of it—it is
the certain grounds of our
daily experience. Chronic
illness is a betrayal of
that fundamental trust"
(Kleinman, 1988, p. 45).*

DISCUSSION OF THE LITERATURE

When faced with cancer, the loss of personal control over one's health can be devastating for many patients. "When I was diagnosed with cancer, my life as I had known it, ended. I was thrown into a life controlled, not by my own will but by doctors, nurses, and technicians. Worst of all, my life was controlled by my disease."

PERCEIVED CONTROL

Control is a multifaceted and complex concept (Thompson & Collins, 1995). An individual's view of, and need for, control appears to be a highly individual and personal matter. There exists a large body of literature on the topic of control that has included various definitions, approaches, and conceptualizations. For the purpose of this discussion within an applied context, the concept of perceived control is discussed with its specific application to situations of medical illness. Perceived control can be defined as the extent to which an individual feels able to obtain good outcomes and avoid undesirable situations as a result of his or her own efforts (Thompson & Collins, 1995).

CONTROL AND COPING

Attempts to delineate the nature of the relationship among individuals' perceptions of control, coping, and subsequent adjustment to illness have yielded inconclusive and contradictory findings (Andrykowski & Brady, 1994). This disparity has been attributed, at least in part, to the complexity of the relationship. Nevertheless, there exists significant evidence that many individuals develop control strategies in response to threatening situations. Traumatic events, such as a cancer diagnosis, can undermine perceived control because the person was not able to exercise control and avoid this serious life event (Thompson & Collins,

1995). Taylor's cognitive adaptation model (Taylor, 1983) hypothesizes that adjustment to a traumatic life event includes three themes: a search for meaning, reestablishment of perceived control or mastery, and the restoration of self-esteem.

CONTROL AND ADJUSTMENT

Subsequent research, much of which has been generated by the Taylor (1983) model, has provided substantial evidence suggesting that those who are able to establish a sense of control will cope better with trauma and experience less associated distress (Affleck, Tennen, & Gersham, 1985; Taylor, Helgeson, Reed, & Skokan, 1991; Thompson, Nanni, & Levine, 1994). Further, perceived control of illness-related events has been associated with better adjustment (Taylor & Spacapan, 1991; Thompson et al.), even in cases of advanced disease (Reed, Taylor, & Kemeny, 1993; Thompson et al.). What appears to be important for adjustment in situations of worsening illness is the shift in control-related beliefs from survival and cure to control of symptoms and life tasks. Thompson et al. make an important distinction between central control, for example, belief that the cancer can be cured, and consequence-related control, believing that the patient can control the consequences of the disease, such as protecting his or her children from upset. In several studies of patients with serious illness, consequence-related control was strongly related to reduced distress, but there was no relationship or only a weak relationship between central control and adjustment (Taylor et al., 1993; Taylor & Collins, 1994). Thus, perceptions of control may continue to be adaptive even when there is only partial truth to them (Taylor et al., 1991).

ILLUSIONS OF CONTROL

In Taylor's (1983) early work, it was hypothesized that perceptions or illusions of control were adaptive to illness adjustment even when they were in clear contradiction to the medical facts. This thinking has been modified somewhat in more recent work to acknowledge that illusions of control are maladaptive when they are in blatant contradiction to existing facts (Taylor et al., 1991; Taylor & Brown, 1994). There is growing agreement that there are limitations to the usefulness of illusions of control, particularly in uncontrollable situations. To be adaptive, control beliefs must be accommodated to the constraints of reality (Taylor & Armor, 1996). It appears that adjustment to illness may be enhanced, at least for some individuals, at mild to moderate levels of perceived control, but the illness–adjustment relationship may break down at high levels of illusion of control (Diener, Colvin, Pavot, & Allman, 1991). Thus, perceptions of control may be adaptive only when there are events that can be controlled, and when that is not possible, it may be preferable for individuals to relinquish personal beliefs of control (Affleck, Tennen, Pfeiffer, & Fifield, 1987; Taylor et al., 1991).

THE DOWNSIDE OF CONTROL

Some investigators have pointed out the burdens associated with personal control. For example, Rodin (1990) notes that having control of a situation places significant demands on individuals, including stress, worry, and self-blame (Rodin, 1986). Despite individuals' desire for control, when perceived that control and its corresponding responsibility are entirely in their hands, individuals may experience heightened distress and search for ways to escape this enormous personal responsibility (Averill, 1973). Recent work with cancer patients lends some support to this argument. Montbriand (1995) has found that control of the cancer situation was seen as too much responsibility for a small subset of patients who accepted full responsibility for control of their illness situation.

VICARIOUS CONTROL

Others chose to give away personal control and thus responsibility to powerful others. For example, Reich and Zautra (1990; 1991) suggest that there are individuals who are better off relying on others for control rather than enhancing their own personal control in stressful situations. However, others have argued that vicarious control, that is, believing that others can exert control, has mixed benefits depending on personal and situational factors, in particular, gender and severity of illness (Taylor et al., 1991). Specifically, these findings indicate that trusting one's physicians with control over illness may be adaptive only for women (Taylor et al., 1984; 1991) and only during early stage disease with well-controlled symptoms and good prognosis (Affleck et al., 1987; Taylor et al., 1991). Thus, it seems that when the disease gets beyond the point of controllability, vicarious control may negatively affect adjustment (Taylor et al., 1991).

THE NEED FOR CONTROL IS RELATIVE

Others point out that the need for personal control is not universal, and some have emphasized the importance of understanding control within its socioeconomic and cultural contexts. For example, Cassileth (1989) notes that the concept of individual autonomy and control, as a distinctly western concept, is considered sacred in the United States. We have a societal tendency "to fill in the gaps of our knowledge in order to rid ourselves of uncertainty, disharmony and the unknown" (p. 1248). In addition, others have suggested that individuals with higher echelon jobs (Lefcourt, 1976) and those with higher levels of education and income (Montbriand, 1995) have greater desire for personal control.

THE NEED FOR CONTROL IS VARIABLE

Moreover, the need for control varies considerably among individuals. As Nunn (1996) notes, there are individual differences in the need for perceived control to feel positively about the future. Further, others suggest that for some individuals, in particular those who are nondefended or self-determinant (Knee & Zuckerman, 1996; 1998), there may exist a much lower need for personal control in stressful situations. Humanistic psychologists have long argued that optimal psychological development is characterized by genuine emotional experiences and by the absence of illusions and psychological defenses (Rogers, 1986). Two recent studies (Knee & Zuckerman, 1996; 1998) lend some support to this line of thinking. Knee and Zuckerman (1996) have found that the use of defensive attributions characterized all individuals except those who possessed personality traits associated with optimal psychological development, providing some support for the idea that "self-determined" individuals exhibit, or perhaps need, fewer distortions, for example control illusions, for self-protection. Similarly, Knee and Zuckerman's (1998) study found that when faced with negative events, self-determined individuals, those oriented toward learning and personal growth, had lower control orientations and used less defensive coping, thus supporting the possibility that individuals with more optimal psychological development may not need illusions when coping with stressful events (Knee & Zuckerman, 1998).

RELINQUISHING CONTROL

Clinically, there is much anecdotal evidence to support the contention that some patients are able to adjust resiliently to illness and relinquish illusions of control with remarkable equanimity. As one patient explained, "I have always believed that my own control over much that happened in my life is greatly limited. That realization has never bothered me. I try to go into each situation both good and bad with an open mind to learn as much as I can, and handle it the best I am able."

In sum, perceptions of control are thought to play a central role in the maintenance of emotional well-being and in the ability to deal successfully with stressful life events. The ability to find control in difficult situations, or maybe more fundamentally the need to find control, may vary considerably among individuals influenced by various personal and contextual factors. Moreover, for certain individuals and in certain situations, relinquishing personal control may provide benefit.

CLINICAL IMPLICATIONS

ASSESSING THE NEED FOR CONTROL

Patients' beliefs about personal control and their need for control are likely to change across the illness trajectory. As clinicians, it is important to assess at various points, particularly at transition points, the benefit–risk ratio of control for our patients. We need to understand the personal meaning of the illness in the context of the patient's culture, religious values, personal beliefs, level of maturity, and personality style.

- Assess the degree of threat to the patient and how disruptive the illness is to the life of the patient.
- What is the patient's need for control?
- How much control does the patient perceive he or she has?
- How much personal control does the patient want?
- Does he or she prefer to rely on staff for control?
- Over what does the patient desire control?
- How distressed is the patient?

In essence, we must know our patients' beliefs and fears to understand their needs for control.

As the poet Ranier Maria Rilke (1986) so eloquently noted, "Our deepest fears are like dragons guarding our deepest treasure" (p. 92).

> Leaving my children is my greatest worry. I have to fight this illness in any way I can. I must live. I will live to see them grown. I'll take the most gruesome treatments, suffer the most horrible side effects, anything to control this cancer. I can't leave them now. They need their mother.

INCREASED THREAT: INCREASED CONTROL

As Folkman (1984) suggests, the greater the appraised threat in a situation, the more important perceptions of control will be. Thus, it is important to understand the psychological distress generated by the threat of the illness. Not only physical threat in terms of disease severity and prognosis, but also personal threat in terms of one's self-concept, personal integrity, and life work. Moreover, when there is a great disparity between expectations for personal control and perceived control, the distress may be heightened.

> I'm a control freak. I expected to have much more control over my life while I was being treated. No one ever told me I wouldn't be able to even get out of bed for the first couple of days after my treatments. This is not what I expected and it makes it all much harder to cope with.

CAUSAL ATTRIBUTIONS TO REGAIN CONTROL

Attribution theorists (Heider, 1958; Weiner, 1985) have suggested that individuals will attribute causes to events to make sense of and gain control over stressful situations. In so doing, individuals will create causal explanations and assign responsibility in various ways, such as by placing blame on themselves or others or by finding external causes to explain stressful situations.

> I know why I got cancer. I never took care of myself. I worked two jobs to support the family while my wife stayed home with the kids. I worked too hard. I played too hard. But now all that is changed, and I know what I have to do to beat this thing.

> I blame my husband for my cancer. I've had nothing but aggravation in my life because of him. This stress made me sick.

INDIVIDUALIZE INTERVENTIONS TO SUPPORT REALISTIC PERSONAL CONTROL

As clinicians, we should facilitate patients' search for personal meaning and understanding of illness within their particular life experience. Listen to personal explanations. Support this reasoning when helpful, but challenge attributions and offer rebuttals when they only add distress.

For some patients, however, the burden of personal control is too great, and they need others to take control of the disease.

> I need my doctors to handle this treatment. I don't want to have to make all these medical decisions. I'm not a doctor. I just want to be told what to do to get better and I will do it.

Taylor et al. (1991) caution that we must be careful when encouraging patients to turn over control to their physicians. This often comes at a cost and may only increase distress and threaten adjustment over time, particularly for those with progressive, uncontrollable disease. Thus, it is important to acknowledge the limits of medical science and of prognostication. Offer support and realistic hope, raise reasonable doubts, and resist making overstated promises.

SPECTRUM OF EMOTIONAL REACTIONS

Expectedly, there will be various responses to the threatened loss of personal control, along with many associated emotions, many of which can be anticipated and all of which need to be assessed. For example, patients may be angry at losing control, and that anger may be directed at family, friends, physicians, and staff. Others may be depressed, anxious, hopeless, frightened. Some may search for meaning and struggle with the questions, "Why me?" "Why at this time in my life?" They may feel guilt and blame themselves, blame others, or blame God for their disease. Others may experience more positive emotions, such as acceptance of the inevitable, viewing their illness as an opportunity for learning and personal growth. Some may experience a deepening of their personal faith and spiritual beliefs, a clarification of the importance of life and of those closest to them, and still others may be relieved to give away the burdens of personal control. If the patient's emotional responses are intense, unrelenting, and disruptive to daily life, refer to mental health professionals for further evaluation and counseling.

WHEN CONTROL IS NEEDED TO MITIGATE DISTRESS

Some patients may not be willing or able to acknowledge the loss of personal control, even when faced with advanced disease. Beliefs in personal control at these times may be serving a very useful purpose in helping to contain the patient's emotional distress. As Taylor et al. (1991) note, perceptions of personal control, even when unrealistic to the state of illness, may be adaptive for some. They caution that viewing perceived control as a state of denial and directly confronting the patient may be misguided and even destructive. In these situations, it becomes important to support the patient's need for control while encouraging necessary planning and problem solving. However, there may be times when, as Taylor and Brown (1988) describe, there exist "windows of realism," during which some patients suspend their illusions in favor of a more realistic view. During these times, be ready to seize the opportunity for frank discussion.

CONTROL COMES AT A COST

There are costs associated with control, particularly with unreasonable control. When possible, we should help patients reduce the burdens of personal control when they become too great and when personal control of the disease becomes unlikely. Do a cost–benefit analysis of control. Guide patients in weighing the advantages and disadvantages associated with personal control. Point out that in uncontrollable situations, illusions of control may create considerable distress and may only set the patient up for added pain by creating false hope, unrealized expectations, and missed opportunities for meaningful communication with loved ones. Over the course of the illness, assist patients with reality checks to help keep their expectations in line with the reality of the illness. As Rodin (1990) notes, engaging in futile attempts at control can cause significant distress. Attempting to control what can't be controlled can be an enormous additional burden for patients. It forces them to use considerable personal resources of time, effort, and energy to maintain these control illusions, and for what gain?

CONTROL WHAT YOU CAN

According to Bandura's cognitive social learning theory (1977), an important component of control is self-efficacy, which can be defined as the expectancy of gaining a good outcome by having personal control. As Thompson and Collins (1995) note, self-efficacy can guide interventions to support behavioral change and enhance control because individuals may underestimate their skills and strengths and need guidance to realize the abilities they possess. Thus, for clinical application, it becomes important to reduce patients' feelings of helplessness as much as possible by offering positive reinforcement, providing information about disease management and symptom management, and maximizing self-care activities. Help patients identify misconceptions, inadequate information, or lack of resources. Enhance patient autonomy by involving patients actively in all relevant decision making.

SHIFT IN FOCUS OF CONTROL

To support patients' self-efficacy, there will be times that patients may need guidance to make the shift from central control to consequence-related control (Thompson et al., 1994). This means altering goals to target those aspects of disease management that are still under the patient's control. This shift may call for various interventions, such as helping patients identify attainable goals for control, teaching patients to use and to modify various techniques for symptom control (eg, pain, nausea, fatigue), helping patients manage their distress and the upset of their loved ones, and assisting them with resource identification, including alternative therapy, mind–body techniques, nutrition teaching, support groups, and counseling. Thus, support patients in various ways to assist them in gaining control over the manageable aspects of their disease and their responses.

CONTROL-ENHANCING STRATEGIES

Additionally, Thompson and Collins (1995) have identified several specific control-enhancing techniques:

- Identify what you want (and are able) to control.
- Identify workable ways to obtain it.
- Switch to alternate goals when original goals are not attainable.
- Recognize your skills and abilities.
- Know how to enhance these skills.
- Decide when trying to assert control is not worth the effort.

In conclusion, expect the need for control to fluctuate depending on the illness course, degree of threat, and distress it creates for the patient. Assist patients to control what they can, when they can, and guide them to relinquish personal control when it is no longer of benefit.

CLINICAL STRATEGIES

1. Respect the dignity and inherent worth of the patient.
2. Be with the patient wherever he or she needs to be psychologically.
3. Compassionately care for patients on their own terms.
4. Guide patients to acknowledge and enhance their personal strengths. Minimize patients' feelings of helplessness.
5. Validate the emotional pain; support the necessary grieving related to loss of control, or positively reframe the situation in response to patient's needs.
6. Understand and respect the patient's coping skills.
7. Recognize the patient's need for control and the purpose it serves during threatening times.
8. Teach new ways of enhancing personal control to those who are receptive to such strategies.
9. Support the patient's need for self-reflection and the creation of personal meaning.
10. Match the patient's need for control with control-enhancing interventions.
11. Offer support to family members as they react to the patient's loss of control and to their own.

CASE STUDY

Loss of control can be a powerful teacher. After a 61-year-old man failed three treatments for liver cancer, he discussed his changing perspective of personal control.

Before I got sick, there was no obstacle that I met that I couldn't overcome. Cancer is the exception. This has been a most humbling experience for me. It is the most painful experience of my life but at the same time, the most enlightening. I've learned so much from being ill. Things I never knew I had to learn. Like giving up my need to control my life and everyone in it. That was always my strength, to solve problems, anticipate obstacles, resolve conflicts, and not let situations get out of hand. Now I'm finding that my need for control is actually the cause of much of my anguish. I won't let my wife help me because I should be able to dress myself. I won't take the pain medications because I should be able to endure my pain without assistance. I won't talk to my friends because I don't want them to see me weak and help-

less. I could go on and on. I am wasting so much energy trying to do battle with every situation, with every symptom, even with every person who cares about me. I've grown weary of fighting. I'm wasting what precious little energy I have left. Now, I'm trying to let go and let people help. I need them now.

REFERENCES

Affleck, G., Tennen, H., & Gersham, K. (1985). Cognitive adaptations to high risk infants: The search for mastery, meaning, and protection from future harm. *American Journal of Mental Deficiency, 89,* 653–656.

Affleck, G., Tennen, H., Pfeiffer, C., & Fifield, J. (1987). Appraisals of control and predictability in adapting to a chronic disease. *Journal of Personality and Social Psychology, 53,* 273–279.

Andrykowski, M. A., & Brady, M. J. (1994). Health locus of control and psychological distress in cancer patients: Interactive effects of context. *Journal of Behavioral Medicine, 17*(5), 439–458.

Averill, J. R. (1973). Personal control over aversive stimuli and its relation to stress. *Psychological Bulletin, 80*(4), 286–303.

Bandura, A. (1977). Self-efficacy: Toward a unifying theory of behavior change. *Psychological Review, 84,* 191–215.

Cassileth, B. (1989). The social implications of questionable therapies. *Cancer, 63*(7), 1247–1250.

Diener, E., Colvin, C. R., Pavot, W. G., & Allman, A. (1991). The psychic costs of intense positive affect. *Journal of Personality and Social Psychology, 61,* 492–503.

Folkman, S. (1984). Personal control and stress and coping processes: A theoretical analysis. *Journal of Personality and Social Psychology, 46,* 839–852.

Heider, F. (1958). *The psychology of interpersonal relations.* New York: Wiley.

Kleinman, A. (1988). *Illness narratives.* New York: U.S. Basic Books.

Knee, C. R., & Zuckerman, M., (1998). A nondefensive personality: Autonomy and control as moderators of defensive coping and self-handicapping. *Journal of Research in Personality, 32*(2), 115–130.

Knee, C. R., & Zuckerman, M. (1996). Causality orientations and the disappearance of the self-serving bias. *Journal of Research in Personality, 30*(1), 76–87.

Lefcourt, H. M. (1976). Locus of control: Current trends in theory and research. Hillsdale, NJ: Lawrence Erlbaum.

Montbriand, M. J. (1995). Alternative therapies as control behaviors used by cancer patients. *Journal of Advanced Nursing, 22,* 646–654.

Nunn, K. P. (1996). Personal hopefulness: A conceptual review of the relevance of the perceived future to psychiatry. *British Journal of Medical Psychology, 69,* 227–245.

Reed, G. M., Taylor, S. E., & Kemeny, M. E. (1993). Perceived control and psychological adjustment in gay men with AIDS. *Journal of Applied Social Psychology, 23,* 791–824.

Reich, J. W., & Zautra, A. J. (1990). Dispositional control beliefs and the consequences of a control-enhancing intervention. *Journal of Gerontology: Psychological Sciences, 45,* 46–51.

Reich, J. W., & Zautra, A. J. (1991). Experimental and measurement approaches to internal control in at-risk older adults. *Journal of Social Issues, 47*(4), 143–158.

Rilke, R. M. (1986). *Letters to young poet.* (S. Mitchell, Trans.). New York: Vintage Books.

Rodin, J. (1986). Aging and health: Effects of the sense of control. *Science, 233*(4770), 1271–1276.

Rodin, J. (1990). Control by any other name: Definitions, concepts, and processes. In J. Rodin, C. Schooler, & K. W. Schaie, (Eds.), *Self-directedness: Cause and effect throughout the life course* (pp. 1–17). Hillsdale, NJ: Lawrence Erlbaum.

Rogers, C. (1986). Carl Rogers on the development of the person-centered approach. *Person-Centered Review, 1*(3), 257–259.

Taylor, S. E. (1983). Adjustment to threatening events: A theory of cognitive adaptation. *American Psychologist, 38,* 1161–1173.

Taylor, S. E., & Armor, D. A. (1996). Positive illusions and coping with adversity. *Journal of Personality, 64*(4), 873–897.

Taylor, S. E., & Brown, J. D. (1994). Positive illusions and well-being revisited: Separating fact from fiction. *Psychological Bulletin, 116*(1), 21–27.

Taylor, S. E., Helgeson, V. S., Reed, G. M., & Skokan, L. A. (1991). Self-generated feelings of control and adjustment to physical illness. *Journal of Social Issues, 47*(4), 91–109.

Taylor, S. E., Wayment, H. A., & Collins, M. A. (1993). Positive illusions and affect regulation. In D. M. Wegner & D. W. Pennebaker (Eds.), *Handbook of mental control* (pp. 325–343). Englewood Cliffs, N. J.: Prentice-Hall.

Thompson, S. C., & Collins, M. A. (1995). Applications of perceived control to cancer: An overview of theory and measurement. *Journal of Psychosocial Oncology, 13*(1/2), 11–26.

Thompson, S. C., Nanni, C., & Levine, A. (1994). Primary versus secondary and disease versus consequence-related control in HIV-positive men. *Journal of Personality and Social Psychology, 67,* 540–547.

Thompson, S. C., & Spacapan, S. (1991). Perceptions of control in vulnerable populations. *Journal of Social Issues, 47*(4), 1–21.

Weiner, B. (1985). An attributional theory of achievement motivation and emotion. *Psychological Review, 42,* 548–573.

This painting was a reaction to the death in January 1998 of my good friend, Dr. Patricia Allison, a retired professor at the University of Pennsylvania. *Throwing Spiders* shows the incredible, rapid explosive advance of her cancer.

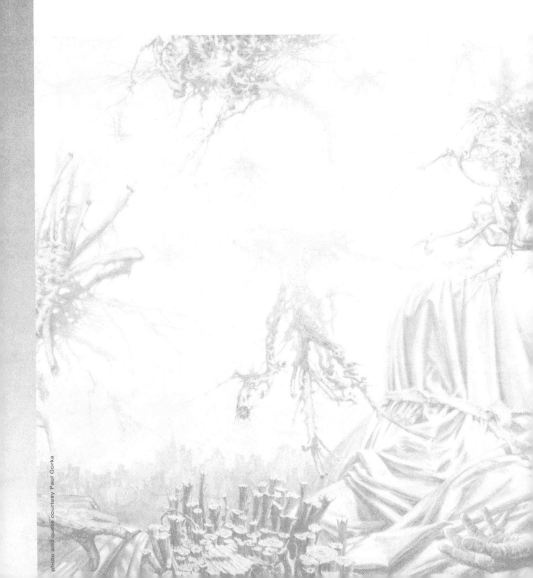

CHAPTER 6

Suffering

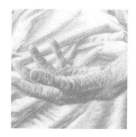

"We must never forget that we may also find meaning in life when confronted with a hopeless situation, when facing a fate that cannot be changed. For what then matters is to bear witness to the uniquely human potential at its best, which is to transform a personal tragedy into triumph, to turn one's predicament into a human achievement. When we are no longer able to change a situation, we are challenged to change ourselves" (Frankl, 1984, p. 15).

DISCUSSION OF THE LITERATURE

When confronted with cancer, there are often many occasions of suffering that can be opportunities for growth or times of great personal anguish. While suffering is associated with situations of illness and is unquestionably a fundamental condition of human nature, it has only recently been accorded legitimacy within the health professions (Cassell, 1992; Morse & Johnson, 1991) and subjected to scientific scrutiny. Traditionally, suffering has been relegated to the religious and to the philosophic, but suffering is now acknowledged as an integral part of the illness experience (Gregory, 1994a). Cassell (1992) suggests that one reason for the dearth of scientific inquiry into the topic of suffering is that the reductive methods of science invariably lead away from an understanding of such a uniquely personal and ubiquitous concept as suffering.

WHAT IS SUFFERING?

Over the years, rich theoretical work has described the experience of suffering. Suffering can be defined as enduring, inevitable, or unavoidable loss; distress; pain; or injury (Pollock & Sands, 1997). Frankl (1984) notes that physical pain and deprivation of themselves are not sufficient to cause suffering. Suffering depends on a personally experienced loss of meaning and purpose. Moreover, Frankl (1984) emphasizes the spiritual dimension of suffering and the power of the human spirit to overcome suffering and in so doing to find new meaning in life. Because suffering is dependent upon the meaning of an event or of a loss for an individual, it cannot be assumed present or absent in any given situation (Kahn & Steeves, 1995). Suffering can only be understood as it is perceived by the person experiencing the suffering (Rodgers & Cowles, 1997).

THE NATURE OF SUFFERING

Suffering has physical, cognitive, affective, social, cultural, existential, and spiritual components (Rodgers & Cowles, 1997). Nevertheless, many theorists point out that suffering defies precise definition because it is a complex subjective phenomenon (Benedict, 1989; Cassell, 1982) and is uniquely experienced by each individual (Graneheim, Lindahl, & Kihlgren, 1997; Eriksson, 1997). "Suffering takes place at the level of the whole person" (Kahn & Steeves, 1995, p. 15). As such, it is a profoundly subjective, holistic experience that is created from the biography and lived world experiences of individuals (Gregory, 1994a). Indeed from a Buddhist perspective, Rinpoche (1994) has observed that suffering in fact has no objective existence. What gives it existence and power over us is only our aversion to it.

Suffering, while an intensely private and personal experience, is at the same time social in nature. As Cassell (1992) noted, "the suffering of the individual is born from shared meanings" (p. 6). It can readily be shared because we all experience suffering. However, the language of suffering is always uniquely personal (Nouwen, 1986; Rodgers & Cowles, 1997).

ISOLATION

Cassell (1992) goes on to observe that the social nature of suffering is highlighted by the isolation imposed by suffering. Suffering forces the individual to focus on the source of the suffering and to withdraw into oneself and away from the world of others. This isolation further adds to the individual's suffering as it disrupts those aspects of a person that require social contact and connection. Suffering people lose their transcendent connection to others. The importance of this loss of transcendence in suffering is suggested by how suffering can be overcome by various transcendent means, such as spirituality (Cassell, 1992).

SELF-CONFLICT

Cassell (1992) also describes the self-conflict that is inherent in suffering. In situations of medical illness, the conflict often centers on the person's beliefs of normal behavior and the demands of the illness. If these struggles are severe enough, the integrity of the person will be threatened, and suffering will follow. This conflict can be depicted as a battle of life purposes in which the person must choose either to maintain one's original purpose, even though it is poorly suited to one's new illness state; develop a new set of life purposes more congruent with a life of chronic illness; or lose a central purpose altogether (Cassell, 1992). "Suffering has as its root sense, the idea of submitting or being forced to submit to some particular set of circumstances, forced to admit to an existence that is not under our control, or to the intrusion of an activity (such as illness) operating under another law than ours. Thus, it is a threat to our autonomy" (Younger, 1995, p. 55).

PERSONAL GROWTH

However, it is by this very threat to identity that personal growth may take shape. A threat to our identity often brings about conditions that are necessary, but not sufficient, for an experience of meaning. These experiences of meaning may alter how one perceives suffering and how one copes with it (Younger, 1995). Suffering "brings one closer to one's own existence because it breaks down the habit and the routine that are great veils, which, when securely in place, allow us not to consider what life means" (Younger, 1995, p.55). Further, both Christian and Buddhist teachings consider suffering an inevitable component of human life, and both identify purpose and potential opportunity for personal growth within the suffering experience (Gregory, 1994a; Rinpoche, 1994).

CONTROLLING SUFFERING: IS IT POSSIBLE?

There may be value in allowing individuals to experience their suffering, find new meaning, let go of what no longer is relevant, and transcend the suffering experience in a strengthened manner. Therefore, we should support the individual in his or her suffering work to embrace, or "befriend," the suffering and asking what one can learn through its experience (Nouwen, 1986; Uomoto, 1995). Suffering work has been described as the work done to move through a situation of pain to a moment of healing (Emerson, 1986) and growth (Frankl, 1984). Moreover, Gregory (1994a) cautions that there are dangers inherent in attempting to control the suffering of others. The quest to control suffering transforms a profoundly complex human experience into essentially a physical condition amenable to treatment. The expectation of control of suffering confers a measure of omnipotence on clinicians. They are in charge of suffering. Suffering is not amenable to control by others. Others may provide conditions that assist a patient to work through or come to terms with their suffering or to provide comfort, but they cannot control a person's suffering (Gregory, 1994a).

INDIVIDUAL INTERPRETATION OF SUFFERING

Suffering has potential value, and both personal goals and beliefs are intimately involved in the individual's interpretation of suffering (Hinds, 1992). Suffering for some may be viewed as a torment, punishment, violation, or as pointless; others may view suffering as inevitable, a source of meaning, a time of learning and growth. The response to the patient should be guided by the individual's description of suffering (Graneheim et al., 1997; Frankl, 1984). The outcome of suffering is ultimately determined by the individual within the context of life experiences, and personal beliefs and values that are brought to bear in the illness situation.

Recent empirical research has focused on the study of the nature and type of suffering correlated with various types of illness (Lindholm & Eriksson, 1993; Kuuppelomaki & Lauri, 1998) and the process of suffering and coping mechanisms (Battenfield, 1984). Findings support the theoretical views that suffering is a uniquely personal matter, dynamic in nature with the intensity varying at different stages of the disease. Most patients find some meaning through their suffering (Kuuppelomaki & Lauri, 1998). For many, suffering can result in personal growth and development (Eriksson, 1997).

SOURCES OF SUFFERING

Some investigators have found that for patients with cancer, the source of physical suffering often lies either in the illness itself or in its treatment (Kuuppelomaki & Lauri, 1998; Cassell, 1992). Further, Gregory (1994b) has found that narrative themes of suffering in individuals with cancer include a cascade of losses, such as undermining of their personhood, failure of treatment as cure, deaths of other cancer patients, and the false reassurance for some that their cancer can be beaten. Other themes include cancer as torture and the beauty of cancer. The patients' suffering was shaped by their past, present, and future experiences. The support of loved ones, faith and trust in God, and satisfaction with life's accomplishments all support patients' endurance of suffering (Gregory, 1994b).

Others (Cherny, Coyle, & Foley, 1994) have identified relevant factors that contribute to the suffering of people with cancer, including physical symptoms, psychological distress, existential concerns, and empathetic suffering with the burdens of their loved ones. Specifically, physical suffering, such as fatigue, pain, and side effects of treatments, and psychological suffering, such as depression, anxiety, loneliness, dependence, helplessness, and fear of death (Kuuppelomaki & Lauri, 1998), are common sources of suffering. The patients' existential distress has been found to include hopelessness, futility, meaninglessness, remorse, and disruption of personal identity (Cassell, 1982; Rowland, 1990).

CHRONIC SORROW

Some individuals with cancer may suffer through their experiences of chronic sorrow. A separate but related line of research has examined the experience of chronic sorrow. Chronic sorrow was first described in 1962 by Olshansky to capture the normal psychological reaction he observed in parents of mentally challenged children. Chronic sorrow can be defined as a pervasive sadness that is permanent, periodic, and progressive (Lindgren, Burke, Hainsworth, & Eakes, 1992). Most of the earlier research focused on parents of children with a mental or physical disability (Hainsworth, 1996). Recently, study of chronic sorrow has expanded to include those with chronic or life-threatening conditions and their caregivers. These studies support the premise that chronic sorrow is likely to occur in various chronic situations that cause a lifestyle disruption (Hainsworth, 1996). The experience of chronic sorrow does not seem to be linked to the length of the illness, but rather to the individual's interpretation of the change and its impact on his or her life situation (Lindgren, 1996). It is a common but not universal experience for patients and their loved ones (Lindgren, 1996). Chronic sorrow can have a deep impact on an individual's sense of self, normalcy, and relationships with others. Chronic sorrow is unresolvable, and further losses and changes may require even greater effort to cope (Lindgren, 1996).

In sum, there is substantial theoretical literature and growing scientific study of suffering in situations of medical illness, including the experience of chronic sorrow, to guide meaningful clinical interventions.

CLINICAL IMPLICATIONS

THE REASONS FOR SUFFERING ARE VARIABLE

It is important for clinicians to recognize that the intensity of suffering from cancer varies widely among patients depending on the form and severity of the disease; the illness course and prognosis; patients' values, beliefs, goals, and aspirations; and the losses and stressors they bring with them into the illness experience.

In my counseling work with patients, I have seen a number of patients whose sources of suffering were related to past issues and current life crises rather than to the illness. For example, for some patients, suffering was caused by childhood abuse, marital problems, grief related to deaths of loved ones, and perceived abandonment by adult children. One patient observed the following:

> It is so foolish and so unexpected to me. All I can seem to think about now is my mother's death. She died when I was 12. How much I miss her and what horrible pain and suffering she must have gone through. I haven't thought much about her for years and years. Now, when I should be worried about my treatments and about fighting my disease, all I seem to be able to do is cry about my mom.

THE PERSONAL CONTEXT OF SUFFERING

It becomes important to meet the patient where he or she is, allowing each patient to move where and when able (Byock, 1994). Each of our patients will suffer differently, for different reasons and purposes. Some will suffer greatly. Some will not suffer at all. Physical illness provides only one aspect of suffering. Some patients may suffer from long-forgotten childhood crises and losses. Others may suffer because of their inability to maintain normalcy in day-to-day living or because of the threatened disruption of future goals and aspirations (eg, the inability to provide for their family, the loss of future opportunities to see their grandchildren, the inability to enjoy retirement, the inability to advance in one's chosen career). We need to understand the patient's personal context of suffering and anticipate that across the course of the illness, the patient's suffering will change in form, intensity, meaning, and context. We need to assess and periodically reassess the patient's experience of suffering to understand his or her physical, psychological, spiritual, and existential issues and needs. Assess the impact of loved ones' suffering on the patient. Ask the patient what is creating the greatest suffering and what the identifiable sources of his or her pain and anguish are.

CARING BY SHARING THE SUFFERING OF PATIENTS

As health care professionals, our response to a patient's suffering is to be with and to care for the patient. The task of confronting the patient's suffering is rightly approached with great humility (Byock, 1994). Sharing a patient's suffering is a gift, a privilege (Gregory, 1994a). We must prove ourselves willing and able to understand the suffering of our patients and then wait for the patients' invitation to share in their suffering, answering it with authentic presence and empathetic caring. Empathetic caring has been beautifully described by Nouwen (1974):

> The word 'care' finds its roots in the Gothic 'Kara' which means lament. The basic meaning of care is: to grieve, to experience sorrow, to cry out with. I am very much struck by this background of the word care because we tend to look at caring as an attitude of the strong toward the weak, of the powerful toward the powerless. Still, when we honestly ask ourselves which persons in our lives mean the most to us, we often find that it is those who, instead of giving much advice, solutions, or cures, have chosen rather to share our pain and touch our wounds with a gentle and tender hand. (pp. 33–34)

WHAT DO PATIENTS WANT FROM CAREGIVERS?

Recent work has described patients' needs while suffering. Patients wish for nurses to have the ability to see behind the symptoms and create a deeper human relationship with their patients. The patients reported a desire for love—longing to be seen, affirmed, and understood—to have their needs met beyond the level of problems. Patients expressed the need for nurses "to partake in the patient's suffering" (Fagerstrom, Eriksson, & Bergbom, 1998, p. 984). Further, Fagerstrom et al. have found that patients will express their needs corresponding to how they view the person of the nurse and based on the patients' judgment of the nurses' ability to understand and fulfill their needs.

RELIEVING SUFFERING

As clinicians, we can have a significant impact on alleviating the suffering of patients by sharing their burdens through understanding the meaning of their suffering. However, it is not as professionals that we meet the sufferer, rather as people who encounter the presence of other people who suffer (Gregory, 1994a). We must control physical symptoms and psychological disorders as well as possible to provide a quiet body and mind, which allows the patient the opportunity to refocus attention on the concerns of the spirit, finding meaning, purpose, forgiveness, and other matters of the heart. However, our goal should not be to control all of the patient's suffering (Gregory, 1994a). As Gregory (1994a) notes, this is an impossible and unreasonable expectation.

LISTEN FROM THE HEART

We need to offer our patients understanding, empathy, and compassion and engage in meaningful communication (Gregory, 1994a) with our patients. Meaningful communication involves the ability to empty oneself and listen (Byock, 1994). As Nouwen (1972) describes, respond to the sufferer from the heart, listen to what the patient is saying, not what you can do with what he or she is saying. Pay attention without personal intention or judgment. This involves intense concentration that requires us to be at peace, settled not restless and conflicted within ourselves. Only then can we create the necessary space for the patient to be himself or herself and come to us on his or her own terms and speak without fear (Nouwen, 1972). While we can't take away all the patient's suffering, we can be present to the patient's suffering, helping him or her shoulder the burdens and find purpose and meaning in a manner congruent with his or her needs and life goals. Thereby, the patient's suffering will be understood, witnessed, and affirmed by clinicians who care enough to go the journey.

COMPASSION

Our understanding should be tempered with compassion. It is important to make a distinction between compassion and pity. As Rinpoche (1994) notes, compassion is a far greater and nobler thing than pity. Pity has its roots in fear and a sense of arrogance. As Stephen Levine says, "When your fear touches someone's pain, it becomes pity; when your love touches someone's pain, it becomes compassion." He observed that to train in compassion is to know that all human beings are the same and suffer in similar ways, to honor all those who suffer, and to know you are neither separate from nor superior to anyone. This relationship with the patient at the level of shared humanity is an exquisitely supportive one. Extending a humane presence to the patient, that is being in tune with the patient's messages (Younger, 1995), enables us to provide existential care to our patients. Existential care can be defined as the compassion and care that are products of the awareness of the common bonds of humanity, common fates, common experiences, and common feelings (Younger, 1995). Caring acknowledgement of patients' suffering legitimizes their experiences and gives patients feelings of wholeness and value (Suchman & Matthews, 1988).

MEANING OF SUFFERING

We need to appreciate that whatever meaning there may be in suffering is for the patient to determine. Guide patients to find purpose and meaning when possible.

A common form for the expression of suffering and search for meaning is the narrative (Younger, 1995). Listen to the patient's story, and support the patient in connecting and developing life themes to create meaning from the suffering experience. Also, help patients transcend suffering through whatever means are acceptable and familiar to them (eg, prayer, meditation, religious or spiritual practices, connections with loved ones). A meditation technique that may be of benefit is described by Rinpoche (1994). It is the Buddhist practice of Tonglen. Tonglen, simply described, is a practice of giving and receiving, taking on the pain and suffering of others and giving them your happiness, well-being, and peace of mind. Specifically, Rinpoche suggests that those who are suffering should be guided to think of all others who are in a pain similar or worse than their own and fill their heart with compassion for them. They should pray to whomever they believe in, asking that their suffering help alleviate the suffering of others. This practice can be helpful in attributing meaning for the pain—to recognize that one's personal suffering is not without meaning and purpose.

LOSS OF CONNECTION

The suffering that accompanies illness may often be compounded by suffering loss of community and connectedness with others (Marris, 1974). This loss of connection may contribute to the isolation and loneliness of the suffering patient (Younger, 1995). Be observant of various reactions that may contribute to the isolation of patients, such as fear, discomfort, and uneasiness of family members, friends, and staff when witnessing patients' suffering. Communicate to loved ones the patient's needs for their presence and support, even if this only involves sitting quietly with the patient. Be aware of the concerns and fears within ourselves as well as in family members, and support and strengthen the bonds between patients and significant others.

INTERVENTIONS FOR PATIENTS WITH CHRONIC SORROW

It is important to distinguish chronic sorrow from depression among the medically ill because the corresponding treatments and interventions would differ. Symptoms that are expected to accompany depression, such as low self-esteem, decreased feelings of self-worth, apathy, negativism, and guilt, would not be seen in cases of chronic sorrow (Lindgren et al., 1992). Chronic sorrow is cyclical and is often triggered by internal or external stimuli that remind the person of their losses (Lindgren et al., 1992). In cases of chronic sorrow, identify trigger events. These may include management crises, such as diagnostic tests, hospitalization, illness recurrence, diagnosis of cancer in friend or family member, or confronting physical reminders of the disease (Eakes, 1993). Chronic sorrow interventions include the following:

- Providing opportunities to discuss fears and concerns
- Communicating information about disease in a timely manner
- Providing anticipatory guidance to patients and family members, explaining the normalcy of experiencing episodes of grief-related feelings (Eakes, 1993)
- Coaching patients and family members on how to talk and listen to one another and recognizing that patients and families may not have the energy and stamina to seek out resources and assistance on their own
- Advocating on their behalf when needed (Krafft & Krafft, 1998)
- Recognizing that prior losses may be exacerbated when dealing with the current losses related to cancer
- Respecting feelings of grief as signals that grief work must be attended to for healthy resolution

Other management strategies include action strategies, such as maintaining involvement in personal interests and activities; cognitive methods, such as reframing; positive attitude and interpersonal techniques, such as support groups and counseling (Eakes, 1993; Hainsworth, 1996).

THE SUFFERING OF THE FAMILY

Another important responsibility for clinicians is to support the suffering of family members. Much support can be indirectly given to families by providing high-quality, compassionate, and dignified care to the patient and by assuring loved ones that all that is possible has been done for the patient. This will go a long way to eliminate additional suffering created by poor care (Brailler, 1992). As much as possible, loved ones should be part of the care team, be involved in relevant decision making, and be kept well-informed of the illness course and the patient's changing needs. Common sources of suffering for caregivers include uncertainty about the future, fear of loneliness, disruption of lifestyle, communication breakdown, helplessness, and lack of support (Hinds, 1992). Hinds (1992) recommends assessing cues that indicate suffering in family members, assisting families to understand and cope constructively with the emotions that contribute to suffering, assisting families to acquire needed information, and correcting suffering-inducing misconceptions. Last, assess adequacy of family supports, and understand and correct discrepancies between what is known and understood by the patient and family (Cherny et al., 1994).

THE SUFFERING OF THE STAFF

The impact of being a witness to the suffering of our patients often creates suffering in physicians, nurses, and oncology staff. This suffering may cause staff to maintain emotional distance, not make time available, and focus exclusively on specific symptoms and their treatment (Klagsbrun, 1994).

The existence of suffering challenges the meaningfulness of our own lives and confronts each of us with our own vulnerability (Cassell, 1982). Recognize that as professional caregivers, we will suffer with our patients. Similar to patients who are attempting to find meaning in their suffering, we as caregivers will suffer less if we continue to find and create meaning in the intense and rewarding work that we have chosen. One of the greatest challenges for us is to initiate and remain in an empathic relationship with patients who are suffering. Doing so allows us to perceive fully the patient's pain and suffering. Remaining open requires considerable expenditure of emotional and spiritual energy, but it allows us to respond with caring approaches that are comforting and effective (Brailler, 1992). Thus, we need to recognize and understand the sources of our own suffering and provide outlets and opportunities for personal support and renewal.

Nouwen (1986) recommends that we suffer with those who suffer but that we do not hold onto the suffering.

> **I believe that I know and share the many sorrows and sad circumstances that a human being can experience, but I do not cling to them. I do not prolong such moments of agony. They pass through me, like life itself, as a broad, eternal stream, they become part of that stream and life continues. (Hillesum, 1984, p. 81)**

CLINICAL STRATEGIES

1. Help patients create a safe physical, psychological, social, and spiritual environment for sustenance and renewal (Brallier, 1992).
2. Be aware of the details and subtleties of the patient's suffering on various dimensions: physical, psychological, social, existential, and spiritual (Brailler, 1992).
3. Aggressively manage symptoms, such as pain, nausea, vomiting, fatigue, sleeplessness, appetite loss, and conditions such as major depression.
4. Listen attentively with empathy and compassion.
5. Support patients' needs for contemplation, reflection, and their search for meaning.
6. Set aside personal preconceptions, and be open to understanding the patient's unique suffering experience (Nouwen, 1986).
7. Recognize that some patients may be less aware than others of what suffering means in their lives (Nouwen, 1986).
8. Help patients come to terms with the purpose and meaning of their suffering in their own style and at their own pace.
9. Listen to the patient's story, to his or her personal account of suffering and its associated meaning.
10. Support patients with their spiritual and existential needs. Refer to counseling and religious or spiritual sources of support as indicated.
11. Provide guidance and support grief work as patients respond to various crises and losses associated with illness and treatment.
12. Support family members in their sorrow and suffering.
13. Take time and care to support yourself on a daily basis because you absorb much of the suffering of your patients.

CASE STUDY

A patient with advanced cancer described his deep suffering and anguish as not resulting from the disease itself but rather from the emotional distance of his wife. The patient observed that he was the "strength" in their relationship. His wife had many needs and many fears. The patient's major concerns were twofold. His wife was not able to be present emotionally and to share his fears and concerns, and his care would become too great a burden for his wife to manage as his disease progressed.

The patient never confided his concerns in a disparaging, critical manner, only as an honest, truthful appraisal of his situation. He didn't want his wife's burdens to be greater than her abilities, but he was "terribly lonely" and felt quite isolated from love and care—at the time of his greatest need.

The patient discussed issues of loneliness, meaning of suffering, death, and struggles with faith in cancer counseling. Goals and a plan of intervention were developed. The oncology staff was apprised of the situation with the intent of putting in place comprehensive home care services to meet the patient's increasing physical needs. His emotional and existential needs were supported through individual counseling and support groups. His wife was supported as well by support groups, counseling, and by the oncology team. The patient expressed feeling understood and supported in his suffering.

REFERENCES

Battenfield, B. L. (1984). Suffering—a conceptual description and content analysis of an operational scheme. *Image: the Journal of Nursing Scholarship, 16*(2), 36–41.

Benedict, S. (1989). The suffering associated with lung cancer. *Cancer Nursing, 12,* 34–40.

Brailler, L. W. (1992).The suffering of terminal illness. In P. L. Starck, & J. P. McGovern (Eds.), *The hidden dimension of illness: Human suffering* (pp. 203–226). New York: National League for Nursing Press.

Byock, I. R. (1994). When suffering persists. *Journal of Palliative Care, 10*(2), 8–13.

Cassell, E. J. (1982). The nature of suffering and the goals of medicine. *New England Journal of Medicine, 306*(11), 639–645.

Cassell, E. (1992). The nature of suffering: Physical, psychological social, and spiritual aspects. In P. L. Starck, & J. M. McGovern (Eds.), *The hidden dimension of illness: Human suffering* (pp. 1–10). New York: National League for Nursing Press.

Cherny, N. I., Coyle, N., & Foley, K. M. (1994). Suffering in the advanced cancer patient: A definition and taxonomy. *Journal of Palliative Care, 10*(2), 57–70.

Eakes, G. G. (1993). Chronic sorrow: A response to living with cancer. *Oncology Nursing Forum, 20*(9), 1327–1334.

Emerson, J. G. (1986). *Suffering: Its meaning and ministry.* Nashville, TN: Abingdon Press.

Eriksson, K. (1997). Understanding the world of the patient, the suffering human being—the new clinical paradigm from nursing to caring. *Advanced Practice Nursing Quarterly, 3,* 8–13.

Fagerstrom L., Eriksson, K., & Bergbom, E. I. (1998). The patient's perceived caring needs as a message of suffering. *Journal of Advanced Nursing, 28*(5), 978–987.

Frankl, V. (1984). *Man's search for meaning.* New York: First Washington Square Press.

Graneheim, U. H., Lindahl, E., & Kihlgren, M. (1997). Descriptions of suffering in connection with life values. *Scandinavian Journal Caring Science, 11,* 145–150.

Gregory, D. M. (1994a). The myth of control: Suffering in palliative care. *Journal of Palliative Care, 10*(2), 18–22.

Gregory, D. M. (1994b). *Narratives of suffering in the cancer experience.* The University of Arizona. Doctoral Dissertation.

Hainsworth, M. A. (1996). Helping spouses with chronic sorrow related to multiple sclerosis. *Journal of Psychosocial Nursing, 34*(6), 36–40.

Hillesum, E. (1984). *The diaries of Etty Hillesum.* New York: Pantheon.

Hinds, C. (1992). Suffering: A relatively unexplored phenomenon among family caregivers of non-institutionalized patients with cancer. *Journal of Advanced Nursing, 17,* 918–925.

Kahn, D. L., & Steeves, R. H. (1995). The significance of suffering in cancer care. *Seminars in Oncology Nursing, 11*(1), 9–16.

Klagsbrun, S. C. (1994). Patient, family, and staff suffering. *Journal of Palliative Care, 10*(2), 14–17.

Krafft, S. K., & Krafft, L. J. (1998). Chronic sorrow: Parents' lived experience. *Holistic Nursing Practice, 13*(1), 59–67.

Kuuppelomaki, M., & Lauri, S. (1998). Cancer patients' reported experiences of suffering. *Cancer Nursing, 21*(5), 364–369.

Lindgren, C. L., Burke, M. L., Hainsworth, M. A., & Eakes, G. G. (1992). Chronic sorrow: A life span concept. *Scholarly Inquiry for Nursing Practice: An International Journal, 6*(4), 27–40.

Lindgren, C. L. (1996). Chronic sorrow in persons with Parkinson's and their spouses. *Scholarly Inquiry for Nursing Practice: An International Journal, 10*(4), 351–366.

Lindholm, L. & Erikson, K. (1993). To understand and alleviate suffering in a caring culture. *Journal of Advanced Nursing, 18,* 1354–1361.

Marris, P. (1974). *Loss and change.* New York: Pantheon.

Morse, J. & Johnson, P. (Eds.). (1991). The illness experience: Dimensions of suffering. Newbury Park: Sage Publications.

Nouwen, H. J. (1972). *The wounded healer.* New York: Image Books Doubleday.

Nouwen, H. J. M. (1974). *Out of solitude: Three meditations on the Christian life.* Notre Dame, IN: Ave Maria Press.

Nouwen, H. J. (1986). *Lifesigns.* New York: Image Books Doubleday.

Olsansky, S. (1962). Chronic sorrow: A response to having a mentally defective child. *Social Casework, 43,* 191–193.

Pollock, S. E., & Sands, D. (1997). Adaptation to suffering. *Clinical Nursing Research, 6*(2) May, 171–185.

Rinpoche, S. (1994). The Tibetan book of living and dying. San Francisco: Harper.

Rodgers, B. L., & Cowles K. V. (1997). A conceptual foundation for human suffering in nursing care and research. *Journal of Advanced Nursing, 25,* 1048–1053.

Rowland, J. H. (1990). Developmental stage and adaptation: Adult model. In J. C. Holland, & J. H. Rowland (Eds.), *Handbook of psychooncology* (pp. 25–43). New York: Oxford University Press.

Suchman, A., & Matthews, D. (1988). What makes the doctor patient relationship therapeutic? Exploring the connexional dimension of medical care. *Annals of Internal Medicine, 108,* 125–130.

Uomoto, J. M. (1995). Human suffering, psychotherapy and soul care: The spirituality of Henri J.M. Nouwen at the nexus. *Journal of Psychology and Christianity, 14*(4), 342–354

Younger, J. B. (1995). The alienation of the sufferer. *Advances in Nursing Science, 17*(4), 53–72.

These photographs were made in Paris,

January 1998, during a break in my treatment at the

Hospital of the University of Pennsylvania.

I wanted to visit a city I worked in

when I was young.

I hope to return.

CHAPTER 7

Meaning of Illness

"The undercurrent of chronic illness is like the volcano: It does not go away. It menaces. It erupts. It is out of control. One damned thing follows another. Confronting crises is only one part of the total picture. The rest is coming to grips with the mundaneness of worries over whether one can negotiate a curb, make it to the bathroom quickly enough, eat breakfast without vomiting, sleep through the night, attempt sexual intercourse, make plans for a vacation, or just plain face up to the myriad of difficulties that make life feel burdened, uncomfortable, and all too often desperate. It has always seemed to me that there is a kind of quiet heroism that comes from meeting these problems and the sentiments they provoke, of getting through each day, of living through the long course with grace and spirit and even humor; sick persons and their families understand the courage, even if most others do not." (Kleinman, 1988, p. 44–45).

DISCUSSION OF THE LITERATURE

The courage to endure an illness such as cancer is often found through the discovery of personal meaning and purpose of the illness. It is an intimate type of meaning that "transfers vital significance from the person's life to the illness experience" (Kleinman, 1988, p. 31). As Frankl (1984) notes, "man's search for meaning is the primary motivation in his life. This meaning is unique and specific in that it must and can be fulfilled by him alone; only then does it achieve a significance that will satisfy his own will to meaning" (Frankl, 1984, p. 121).

PERSONAL MEANING

Over the years, meaning has been examined from various perspectives, among them anthropology, psychology, sociology, and philosophy. These varied approaches inform our current thinking in substantive and diverse ways. While there are various definitions of meaning corresponding to the particular areas of study, there is general agreement that meaning is a central aspect of human existence that is dynamic and changes over time as changes occur in the individual, in illness events, and in the social context (Frankl, 1984; Kleinman, 1988; Fife, 1994). Although the emphasis varies, meaning often refers to the individual's sense of purpose and identity in relation to the world of objects, events, and relationships (Cassell, 1982; Frankl, 1984). The development of personal meaning is influenced by many factors, such as religion, sociocultural background, family, education, personal values and beliefs, and coping style. Disease-related factors include stage, prognosis, and so on (Lipowski, 1970; Luker, Beaver, Leinster, & Owens, 1996). To date, as Fife (1994) has noted, there has been little study of the impact of personal meaning on coping, behavior, and adaptation to illness.

THE SEARCH FOR MEANING

Thompson and Janigian (1988) distinguish between meaning and the search for meaning when one is confronted with stressful life events. They have observed that the search for meaning is part of the coping process, but "found meaning," that is, discovering meaning of personal significance, is a positive aspect of the coping outcome.

Attribution research has contributed significantly to our understanding of the search for personal meaning. Heider's (1958) view that individuals attribute causes to events to make sense of them and to gain control over their lives has served as the basis for attributional theory. Causal thinking, asking "Why did this happen," is the underlying cognitive activity (Lowery & Houldin, 1996). The basic assumptions of causal thinking are that individuals search for causes to interpret new information. Causal thinking is the first step in coping with unexpected life events, and affect, expectations, and actions are based on the causes or personal explanations generated through this search (Weiner, 1985; 1979; Lowery & Houldin, 1996). There has been much study generated by attribution theory with mixed results. Of particular relevance for this discussion is that the attributional search is by no means universal. While some engage in a search to find meaning when faced with illness (Germino, Fife, & Funk, 1995), there is evidence that others do not (Lowery, Jacobsen, & McCauley, 1987; Taylor, Lichtman, & Wood, 1984). Also, there is some evidence that those who do not search for causes of their illness are less distressed than those who do search (Lowery et al., 1987). Further, some research with patients with cancer has not supported a relationship between a search for meaning and improved adjustment to illness (Lowery, Jacobsen, & Ducette, 1993).

THE OUTCOME OF THE SEARCH

Perhaps the efficacy of the search is dependent upon the outcome. Thus, if significant meaning is discovered through the causal search and it helps to explain the illness situation in a manner that does not threaten the identity or integrity of the individual, then most likely the search will be adaptive (Thompson & Janigian, 1988). The primary reason for the search is the desire for a sense of congruence between self-identity and the events, such as illness, that occur (Marris, 1974; Thompson & Janigian, 1988). Therefore, for some individuals, but not for all, critical life events, such as cancer, require that they reconstruct and transform the meaning on which they have based their lives to accommodate the illness event (Fife, 1994). This occurs in response to the many threats that illness can pose to individuals; significant among them are threats to personal control, self-esteem, and body image and threats to the assumptions one holds about life and one's place in the world. Thus, the perceived meaning of the illness will be constructed on the basis of what has been important within the life of each person as he or she is affected by the illness experience (Fife, 1994). It follows that whatever meanings individuals assign to the illness will subsequently influence their coping strategies, behaviors, and actions (Fife, 1994; Lipowski, 1970).

PERSONAL MEANING AND OUTCOMES

Recent research has found that individuals who are able to maintain a positive perspective on themselves and their futures while living with serious illness are able to minimize emotional distress (Fife, 1994); that finding a sense of purpose outside oneself is associated with adaptive coping (O'Connor et al., 1990; Coward, 1991); and that those who cannot find meaning or only find negative meaning are more likely to be distressed and have difficulty adapting to stressful life events than those who can find positive meaning (Wortman & Silver, 1992). Frankl (1984) has observed that when an individual's search for meaning is successful, it gives him or her greater capability to cope with suffering.

Because serious illness is a uniquely personal experience, it is the individual's decision, some say it is the individual's responsibility (Frankl, 1984), as to whether the illness holds personal meaning. "Meaning in life is hard won to the extent that it is within persons' control at all, and it is possible to die having failed to find it or even having failed to recognize the urgency of seeking it" (Attig, 1989, pp. 366–367). Thus, for those who search for meaning when faced with illness, the struggle is to find meaningful answers or to find the means to live without answers (Attig, 1989).

MEANING IS RELATIVE

What constitutes meaningful answers varies among individuals and often within individuals over time. For some, positive meaning may be found in seeing the illness as a challenge to overcome or as an opportunity for growth. For others, taking comfort in religious or spiritual beliefs will provide positive meaning and solace. Both Christian and Buddhist teachings emphasize the importance of "looking within" through prayer and meditation for answers and truth (Bible; Rinpoche, 1994).

FACING MORTALITY

For those with advanced disease in particular, searching for meaning in situations of illness may involve confronting their own mortality. As Attig (1989) has observed, given our cultural patterns of denial and avoidance of personal mortality, "the prospect of our own mortality is not easily taken in" (p. 383). Further, Kleinman (1988) has noted that the North American culture of personal freedom and the pursuit of happiness has come to mean for many guaranteed freedom from pain and suffering. Thus, finding meaning and purpose in illness may involve personal grieving; a self-mourning over lost illusions, assumptions, hopes, and dreams; and coming to terms with one's own fragility and mortality (Attig, 1989). There may be a deep personal anguish and grief over "the death of the person he or she was or hoped to become" (Lewis, 1989). However, successful resolution of this grief often results in a readaptation to life that includes the limitations of the illness (Stephenson & Murphy, 1986) and the realization of the "irreversibility of our lives" (Frankl, 1984). This process can be self-transforming and may hold many benefits, such as a fuller appreciation of life's preciousness, value, and meaning.

WHEN MEANING IS NEGATIVE OR NONEXISTENT

If individuals cannot find any meaning in their illness, they may experience an "existential vacuum," with feelings of depression, emptiness, bitterness, distress, and meaninglessness (Frankl, 1984; Attig, 1989). Similarly, those who search and find only negative meaning, such as viewing the illness as a punishment, a weakness, or an enemy, often experience heightened distress and may have difficulty coping with the illness (Barkwell, 1991).

Thompson and Janigian (1988) have asserted that if individuals cannot find meaning in the illness by changing their former beliefs about themselves and their lives, they may accommodate by changing their perceptions of the illness event itself. Individuals may use cognitive and behavioral strategies, such as avoidance, denial, emotional distancing, positive reframing, or cognitive shifting to focus on diet modification and exercise, in an attempt to minimize the significance of the disease and to protect the validity of what has been the reality of their world (Pfost & Stevens, 1989; Fife, 1994).

PERSONAL WEB OF MEANING

Meaning is a dynamic phenomenon that will often change with time. Serious illness has a deeply private significance, and individuals will likely create their own web of meaning that links the illness experience to the values of one's life world (Kleinman, 1984). Meaning may be implicit for some, and explicit for others. Because people respond to an event based on the particular meanings they have assigned to it, the meaning of the illness event becomes foundational for subsequent coping and behavioral responses (Blumer, 1969; Frazier & Garvin, 1996).

CLINICAL IMPLICATIONS

ILLNESS AS A PROBLEM OF MEANING

As clinicians, it is important to assess illness as potentially "a problem of meaning" (McGrath, 1998) for our patients. Various questions may be useful as an assessment guide to help us understand our patients' view of their illness. For example, some questions include the following:

- Tell me what has changed for you as a result of your illness?
- Have your relationships with family members, friends, coworkers been altered?
- How has the illness affected your self-concept, that is, how you feel about yourself, your appearance, your abilities, your contributions?
- How do you view your illness?

- How disruptive has it been to you?
- How disruptive do you think it may be in the future?
- What gives your life meaning—both now and before the cancer?
- How has your life changed since your diagnosis?
- Which of these changes has been most difficult for you?
- Do you struggle with questions about why you have this illness and why at this time in your life? If so, are you able to find satisfying answers to these questions?
- What helps you to cope with your illness?
- What makes coping more difficult?

PERSONAL MEANING OF CANCER

As a result of the assessment, we can learn a great deal about our patients: Some patients will search and find positive meaning in their illness, and others may be just too frightened to look. When the personal meaning of the illness is known, it is possible to better understand the patient's actions and responses to illness (McGrath, 1998) and how disruptive the illness has been to previous meanings or life themes of importance to the patient (Fife, 1994).

Frankl (1984) has identified in his theory of "logotherapy" three major sources of meaning in people's lives—work, love, and, perhaps most importantly, self-learning and self-growth. It is important for us to understand how these central sources of life meaning have been affected by the patient's illness. Some patients may view cancer as a tormentor, as a teacher, or as a curse. Some patient excerpts are illustrative of these varying perspectives:

> Since I've been sick I found out what's really necessary and who really cares about me. I now understand what and who are important in my life.

> My appearance is most important in my world. You see I'm a model and it may seem superficial to others, but this is my livelihood—my life, who I am. If I don't look good, all that I have worked for my entire life is left in ruins.

> Cancer is a blessing. I no longer worry about what people think of me, what I should be doing to please others. Now, my focus is on being true to myself and doing all I can in my own way whether others like it or not. My time here is short and precious. I don't intend to waste it anymore.

This illness is just a blip, a passing annoyance. I try not to think too much about it and not let it interfere with my life. Just grin and bear it; it will be over soon and then I can get back to my old self.

I don't like to talk about my illness. I don't even look in the mirror, or look at my scar. I just keep an old picture of me up on the refrigerator and think that is me and I refuse to think otherwise.

I get so angry when people say there is a reason for my illness. Every cloud has a silver lining. I could just scream. There is absolutely nothing to be gained from being sick, only heartache and pain.

It is not fair that I'm sick. I'm only 45 years old. I should have many, many more healthy years ahead of me. This is just not as my life was supposed to be.

My faith carries me through this treatment. I am surprised at how well I have done—I credit it all to my trust in God.

Cancer to me is a death sentence. I've worried my whole life . . . I've always been afraid of getting cancer. I feel that now by having this cancer—I am being punished for my past deeds, bad choices, and poor judgment.

Thus, those who do in fact search for meaning find positive or negative meaning, while others find no meaning at all for their illness. Patients will often assign different meanings at different points across the illness trajectory. Some may hold multiple meanings about their illness, for example, challenge and enemy or teacher and impending death.

PERSONAL MEANING AS A DYNAMIC PROCESS

Corresponding to the meanings assigned to the illness, individuals may experience a myriad of feelings: sadness, loneliness, alienation, hopefulness, fear, anxiety, anger, hopelessness, gratitude, guilt; the perceptions of threat, vulnerability, loss of control, powerlessness, and insignificance; a comfort in their faith and beliefs; or an appreciation for a life well-lived. These emotions will ebb and flow and vary in intensity over the course of the illness. Individuals may have difficulty sorting out their emotions to recognize the sources of their upset and to see that some of their feelings may be in response to the perceived threat of illness to one's very existence (Attig, 1989).

SUPPORTING THE DISCOVERY OF PERSONAL MEANING

It is important for us to guide patients to sort out the reasons for their upset, which are often generated by multiple sources—emotional distress, physical distress, existential distress, spiritual distress, and social distress—to put in place meaningful goals, interventions, and support. For example, physical pain or emotional distress may prevent patients from confronting the existential and spiritual issues of importance to them. Thus, we need to disentangle the various causes of patients' distress, treat psychological disturbances and physical distress with appropriate pharmacological and medical interventions, and provide support for patients to explore issues of concern to them, with referrals to spiritual or religious counseling as indicated. As Mathieson and Stam (1991; 1995) have observed, psychosocial oncology would be well served to put less emphasis on diagnosis and classification of psychosocial difficulties and greater emphasis on understanding the lived experience of a chronic, potentially life-threatening illness. Clearly, both are important.

Because patients' styles of coping will depend in large measure on the meanings that cancer holds for them, understanding the meanings assigned to the illness may provide some indication of patients' adjustment to the disease. That is, the more positive the meaning constructed by the individual, the more positive the general psychological adjustment and the adjustment to the illness may be. When individuals view their illness from a highly negative perspective with great anxiety and without hope, it's important to monitor this attitude with ongoing assessments, identify particular sources of distress, offer support, manage symptoms of distress, and make referrals for psychosocial intervention as warranted (Germino et al., 1995).

AUTHENTIC PRESENCE

Several useful interventions have been identified in the literature that can be instructive to clinical practice. Kleinman (1988) notes that clinicians need to be able to "grasp behind the simple sounds of bodily pain and psychiatric symptoms, the complex inner language of hurt, desperation, and the moral pain (and also triumph) of living an illness" (pp. 28–29). Patients need the authentic presence of others who are not afraid to care from the heart and get involved enough to understand their pain.

Kleinman (1988) describes the importance of empathetic witnessing, that is, the existential commitment to be with the patient and offer support as he or she comes to terms with the illness experience in a uniquely individual manner. He makes other recommendations for clinicians:

- Practical coping with the major psychosocial crises that accompany chronic illness
- Sensitive solicitation of the patient's and family's stories of the illness, assembling of a miniethnography of the changing contexts of the illness
- Informed negotiations with the lay perspective on their medical care
- Brief medical crisis counseling for the multiple ongoing threats and losses that make chronic illness so disruptive
- Psychosocial counseling as necessary to support patients to understand and alter meanings that are causing distress
- Alternate meanings provided to patients that fit within their world view; for example, challenge versus obstacle, living versus preparing to die, opportunity versus crisis
- Guidance for patients to incorporate their illness as a meaningful part of their life experiences

PERSONAL STORIES

Meanings that patients attribute to illness are often embedded in the stories they create and tell (Seaburn, Lorenz, & Kaplan, 1992).

> For cancer patients, . . . stories have a special meaning. In negotiating their way through regimens of treatment, changing bodies, and disrupted lives, the telling of one's own story takes on a renewed urgency. In the end, they are more than just stories but the vehicle for making sense of, not just an illness, but a life. (Mathieson & Stam, 1995, p. 284).

Thus, it is important for us to listen to patients' stories and to affirm and value their meanings. Talking, taping, and journaling are various ways for patients to tell their stories.

GRIEF WORK

Moreover, illness to some may mean impending death or the threatened loss of long-cherished goals, dreams, and enduring beliefs. Coming to terms with the realities of the disease, one's personal fragility, and mortality will often involve grieving (Attig, 1989). Further, many individuals hold the world view beliefs that the world is orderly, comprehensible, predictable, and controllable (Zlatin, 1995). The pervasive impact of lost assumptions and illusions associated with serious illness can shake the very foundations of self-understanding and orientation to the world and pose significant challenges to personal integrity and perceived meaningfulness (Attig, 1989).

We must support patients in their grief work, because grieving is essentially the process of finding appropriate meanings (Attig, 1989). Grief work becomes important to patients to mourn anticipated or actual losses and to replace them with new meanings and purposes. For example, a patient may not be able to work any longer to support his family, but he can use his newfound time to read with his children and tell them stories about his life, about their grandparents, and their family legacy. Nonetheless, it is important for patients to understand that finding meaning in illness doesn't necessarily mean an end to their grief, but it can provide an understanding of its purpose.

SUPPORTING MEANINGFUL CONNECTIONS

Because self-transcendence, that is, giving oneself to a cause, belief, or to a loved one, can create meaning, reduce distress, and help the patient to find meaning (Frankl, 1984), it's useful to assist patients to connect to that which is meaningful in their lives. This can include strengthening relationships and bonds with significant others or pets; finding purpose in personal beliefs or work activities, through faith, prayer, or meditation exercises; or by finding opportunities to help others. Support patients through the process of personal reflection, contemplation, and self-understanding. Some patients may look to philosophy, religion, spirituality, or poetry to provide direction and answers.

Altered personal meanings can change a patient's relationships with significant others whose own life meanings and perspectives have not changed or have changed in very different ways. These differences can place strain on interpersonal relationships and change a previously shared sense of purpose with others. Each family member must face changed meaning as a direct result of the patient's illness (Fife, 1994); thus, it's important to support patients and their loved ones as they struggle with changed lives and changed meanings. Keep the lines of communication open and the interpersonal connections as strong as possible.

UNCONDITIONAL PERSONAL WORTH AND VALUE

No matter how devastating and incapacitating the illness may become, it is critical that patients understand that they have intrinsic value that the disease can never take away. As Frankl (1984) notes, life offers each of us unconditional meaning; life remains potentially meaningful under any conditions, paralleled by the unconditional value of each and every person. It is imperative that clinicians and family members convey respect and acknowledge the dignity of the patient at all stages of illness.

USE OF AVOIDANCE STRATEGIES

While some patients may search for personal meaning within themselves or in their lives, others may alter their perceptions of their illness to make sense of the situation and to filter unacceptable meanings (Fife, 1994). Some patients may use avoidance strategies, such as minimizing the seriousness of the illness, downward comparison, and emotional distancing, to avoid confronting the realities of the disease. We need to understand patients' coping strategies as they relate to the meanings they have assigned to their illness and support patients as they find their own best ways of defining and coping with cancer.

OUR CLINICAL REALITY

It's important to appreciate that as clinicians, we have the power to influence our patients' perceptions of illness (Fife, 1994). Additionally, we interpret patients' accounts through our own personal, cultural, and social filters. As Kleinman (1986) notes, "health professionals, when they stop to think about it, recognize that how they listen to these (patient's) accounts constrains the telling and the hearing. All attend differently. The way they nod their head, fidget, or look at the patient influences how the patient tells the illness story" (p. 52). He goes on to label this process as the "clinical reality," that is, the clinician's interpretation of the problem, which may differ significantly from the patient's view of the illness. Kleinman challenges us to "unpack our own interpretive schemes" filled with personal and cultural biases and rethink the versions of the clinical world that we create (p. 53).

THE NEED FOR PERSONAL REFLECTION

This rethinking involves our own reflection and appraisal of how our "world view" may impact on our patients and may potentially interfere with our clinical vision and efficacy. Holding an incomplete or inaccurate picture of the "clinical problem" by not understanding the meanings that cancer holds for our patients can impede effective care.

As caregivers, we need to be aware of our own beliefs about illness and mortality, discovering and developing personal meanings and values and deliberately articulating our own styles in facing illness. This will lead to a deeper appreciation of the grief facing our patients and a deeper understanding and respect for the humanity we all share (Attig, 1989).

CLINICAL STRATEGIES

1. Respect the individuality of each patient by understanding the personal meaning of his or her illness.
2. Provide individualized interventions matched with patients' personal meaning of illness and coping style.
3. Understand that meaning is a dynamic process. Anticipate changes over time. Encourage using the illness event as an opportunity for personal growth.
4. Appreciate that patients' life themes may serve as filters for reinterpreting illness events so that the illness is congruent with long-held beliefs and these themes will help explain the coping strategies that patients use (Zlatin, 1995).
5. Assist patients to find positive meaning, such as taking comfort in a life well lived, their legacy, and accomplishments, in the love they have given and received, or in their beliefs and faith.
6. Support patients' connections to the people, goals, beliefs, and events that are most meaningful to them.
7. Witness the patient's life story, validate its interpretation, and affirm its value (Kleinman, 1986).
8. Support patients in their grief work to resolve illness-related changes, and incorporate losses into their personal context of lived life experiences.
9. Recognize that patients' meanings of illness can be influenced by significant others in their social context, including health professionals (Fife, 1994).

CASE STUDY

A 55-year-old woman with recently diagnosed stage II breast cancer viewed her illness as a teacher. She was a person of deep faith, grateful for a "life filled with blessings," open to whatever she could learn through this personal experience with illness, and willing to be of help to others. The patient came to counseling because, despite her understanding of the meaning and purpose of her illness, she was quite distressed. The patient was concerned about the depth of her sadness. The emotional distress for her was centered on the losses related to altered body image and threats to her self-esteem and self-worth associated with her recent diagnosis, surgery, and treatment. The patient was relieved to hear that her distress was normal, an expected reaction to changes to her identity. After brief medical crisis counseling, her distress diminished significantly as the patient through grief work was able to identify her feelings and begin to come to terms with her losses on an emotional level.

REFERENCES

Attig, T. (1989). Coping with mortality: An essay on self-mourning. *Death Studies, 13,* 361–370.

Barkwell, D. P. (1991). Ascribed meaning: A critical factor in coping and pain attenuation in patients with cancer related pain. *Journal of Palliative Care, 7,* 5–14.

Blumer, H. (1969). *Symbolic interaction: Perspective and method.* Englewood Cliffs, NJ: Prentice-Hall.

Cassel, E. (1982). The nature of suffering and the goals of medicine. *New England Journal of Medicine, 306,* 639–645.

Coward, D. D. (1991). Self-transcendence and emotional well-being in women with advanced breast cancer. *Oncology Nursing Forum, 18,* 857–863.

Fife, B. L. (1994). The conceptualization of meaning in illness. *Social Science Medicine, 38*(2), 309–316.

Frankl, V. E. (1984). *Man's search for meaning.* New York: Washington Square Press.

Frazier, S. K., & Garvin, B. J. (1996). Cardiac patients' conversations and the process of establishing meaning. *Progress in Cardiovascular Nursing, 11*(4), 25–34.

Germino, B. B., Fife, B. L., & Funk, S. G. (1995). Cancer and partner relationships: What is its meaning? *Seminars in Oncology Nursing, 11*(1), 43–50.

Heider, F. (1958). *The psychology of interpersonal relations.* New York: Wiley.

Kleinman, A. (1988). *The illness narratives: Suffering, healing, and the human condition.* New York: Basic Books.

Lewis, F. M. (1989). Attributions of control, experienced meaning, and psychosocial well-being, in patients with advanced cancer. *Journal of Psychosocial Oncology, 7,* 105–119.

Lipowski, Z. (1970). Physical illness, the individual and coping processes. *Psychiatric Medicine, 1*(2), 91–102.

Lowery, B. J., & Houldin, A. D. (1996). From stressor to illness. In A. B. McBride, & J. K. Austin (Eds.), *Psychiatric-mental health nursing: Integrating the behavioral and biological sciences* (pp. 11–29). Philadelphia: W.B. Saunders.

Lowery, B. J., Jacobsen, B., & Ducette, J. (1993). Attributions, control and adjustment to breast cancer. *Psychosocial Oncology, 10*(4), 37–53.

Lowery, B., Jacobsen, B., & McCauley, K., (1987). On the prevalence of causal search in illness situations. *Nursing Research, 36,* 88–93.

Luker, K. A., Beaver, K., Leinster, S. J., & Owens, R. G. (1996). Meaning of illness for women with breast cancer. *Journal of Advanced Nursing, 23,* 1194–1201.

Marris, P. (1974). *Loss and change.* New York: Random House.

Mathieson, C. M., & Stam, H. J. (1991). What good is psychotherapy when I'm ill? Psychosocial problems and interventions with cancer patients. In C. L. Cooper, & M. Watson (Eds.), *Cancer and stress: Psychological, biological and coping studies* (pp. 171–196). Chichester: John Wiley and Sons.

Mathieson, C. M., & Stam, H. J. (1995). Renegotiating identity: Cancer narratives. *Sociology of Health and Illness, 17*(3), 283–306.

McGrath, B. B. (1998). Illness as a problem of meaning: Moving culture from the classroom to the clinic. *Advances in Nursing Science, 21*(2), 17–29.

O'Connor, A. P., Wicker, C. A., & Germino, B. B. (1990). Understanding the cancer patient's search for meaning. *Cancer Nursing, 13,* 167–175.

O'Connor, A. P., & Wicker, C. A. (1995). Clinical commentary: Promoting meaning in the lives of cancer survivors. *Seminars in Oncology Nursing, 11*(1), 68–72.

Pfost, K. S., & Wessels, A. B. (1989). Relationship of purpose in life to grief experiences in response to the death of a significant other. *Death Studies, 13,* 371–378.

Rinpoche. (1993). *The Tibetan book of living and dying.* San Francisco: Harper.

Seaburn, D. B., Lorenz, A., & Kaplan, D. (1992). The transgenerational development of chronic illness meanings. *Family Systems Medicine, 10*(4), 385–394.

Stephenson, J. S., & Murphy, D. (1986). Existential grief: The special case of the chronically ill and disabled. *Death Studies, 10,* 135–145.

Taylor, S. E., Lichtman, R. R., & Wood, J. L. (1984). Attributions, beliefs about control, and adjustment to breast cancer. *Journal of Personality and Social Psychology, 46,* 489–502.

Thompson, S., & Janigian, A. (1988). Life themes: A framework for understanding the search for meaning. *Journal of Social Clinical Psychology, 7*(213), 260–280.

Weiner, B. (1979). A theory of motivation for some classroom experiences. *Journal of Educational Psychology, 71,* 3–25.

Weiner, B. (1985). An attributional theory of achievement motivation and emotion. *Psychological Review, 42,* 548–573.

Wortman, C. B., & Silver, R. C. (1992). Reconsidering assumptions about coping with loss: An overview of current research. In L. Montada, S. Filipp, et al. (Eds.), *Life crises and experiences of loss in adulthood* (pp. 341–365). Hillsdale, NJ: Lawrence Erlbaum Associates.

Zlatin, D. M. (1995). Life themes: A method to understand terminal illness. *Omega, 31*(3), 189–206.

Now approaching my 56th year, I was faced with the threat of serious illness—a cancer diagnosis. During the first spring, I began to paint Easter lilies, the kind that bloom pink and white, the perfume so heavy, enlivening every fiber of my being. I understood the meaning of these lilies, more clearly than ever before: Life, death and rebirth, regeneration, transition, and the beginning and celebration of a journey. These flowers, from Bouquet, were sent to me in the hospital. This was the first painting I did of my experience. I loved the colors and vibrancy of them.

CHAPTER 8

Forgiveness

"The old law of 'an eye for an eye' leaves everybody completely blind"
(Martin Luther King, Jr.).

"If we could read the secret history of our enemies, we should find in each man's
life sorrow and suffering enough to disarm hostility"
(Henry Wadsworth Longfellow).

"When you are offended at any man's fault, turn to yourself and study your
own failings. Then you will forget your anger" (Epictetus).

"To err is human. To forgive is divine" (Alexander Pope).

DISCUSSION OF THE LITERATURE

Forgiveness has a rich history in both religious and philosophical contexts. Recently, forgiveness has been studied in the psychological literature (Enright & Human Development Study Group, 1996) both theoretically and empirically. However, very limited work has been done in understanding forgiveness in medically ill populations. As a result of the existing research, there is some evidence that forgiving may reduce depression, anxiety, and anger (Fitzgibbons, 1986; Kaplan, 1992); help resolve relational conflicts (Davenport, 1991; Hebl & Enright, 1993; Worthington & DiBlasio, 1990); and be valuable in the treatment of post-traumatic stress disorder (Johnson, Feldman, Lubin, & Southwick, 1995) for victims of abuse (Farmer, 1989; Davenport, 1991) and incest (Freedman & Enright, 1996). Additionally, the importance of empathy has been explicated in the forgiving process (McCullough, Worthington, & Rachal, 1997), as has the use of attribution retraining in forgiveness therapy (Al-Mabuk, Dedrick, & Vanderah, 1998).

AN INTEGRATED CONCEPT OF FORGIVENESS

As the concept of forgiveness gains acceptance and use in clinical psychology, Meek and McMinn (1997) have cautioned against the "uncoupling of religion and forgiveness" and the need to understand forgiveness within its philosophical and theological foundation. They point out that a loss of connection overlooks a progression of healing that both includes and transcends personal healing for the forgiver and may weaken the therapeutic efficacy of forgiveness. Thus, the forgiveness process has philosophical, spiritual, and psychological aspects that must be integrated. The central idea of forgiveness therapy is that forgiveness produces an inner adjustment, a change in perspective, through which one sees that there are no real grounds for condemnation of oneself, another person, or a thing. Hurt and anger can thus be changed into a means of finding a more peaceful, less judgmental reality (Phillips & Osborne, 1989).

INDIVIDUAL DIFFERENCES IN FORGIVENESS

There are important individual differences and complexities in forgiving (McCullough et al., 1997). Pingleton (1997) has noted that it is a fundamental axiom of human existence that everyone experiences pain, trauma, and suffering in life, often within the rubric of one's closest interpersonal relationships. Thus, forgiveness is necessitated whenever one sustains a violation of one's sense of fairness or justice or experiences a deprivation of love. Forgiveness is in large measure influenced by many individual factors, such as differences in maturational status, personality style, or psychopathological states. Thus, it is important to conceptualize forgiveness as a "multifaceted process rather than as a simplistic, unitemporal event" (Pingleton, 1997, p. 404).

WHAT IS FORGIVENESS?

While forgiveness in all of its complexity defies definition (Haber, 1991), there are various ways to characterize relevant aspects of forgiveness. For example, forgiveness has been viewed as a conflict-resolution process (Droll, 1984); as a sign of self-respect because forgiveness involves accurately seeing and acknowledging hurt and injustice (Holmgren, 1993); as a function of acceptance and absorption of pain, which is at the heart of forgiveness (Enright & Human Development Study Group, 1996); and as a complicated intrapsychic and interpersonal process that may involve years of effort (Benson, 1992).

FORGIVENESS AS A THERAPEUTIC EVENT

Ritzman (1987) describes forgiveness as a therapeutic event of particular power and importance and the nature of forgiveness as unconditional, always present in relationships of genuine love and in relationships with God, and necessary to heal deep emotional wounds. He emphasizes that forgiveness is necessary not for the sake of the person to be forgiven, but for one's own sake. Further, Enright (1996) notes that forgiveness is always a personal choice, whether it is based on the philosophical grounds, that act in self-respect and human concerns; religious grounds, that as we are able to forgive others, so shall we be forgiven; or psychological grounds, that of improved psychological health by those who are able to forgive. However, forgiveness is not condoning, excusing, forgetting, or tolerating of personal violations or injustices, and it does not necessitate reconciliation (Augsburger, 1981; Benson, 1992; Enright & Human Development Study Group, 1996; Stoop, 1991). Further, forgiveness is not a quick substitute for hate, and denial and repression work against forgiveness by short-circuiting the necessary phase of being in touch with the personal anger and resentment (Benson, 1992) before forgiveness can be given.

SELF-FORGIVENESS

While most of the recent work has centered on interpersonal forgiveness, specifically forgiving others, there has been some examination of the related areas of self-forgiveness and receiving forgiveness from others (Enright & Human Development Study Group, 1996). Self-forgiveness is viewed as the most difficult of these, because most individuals are harder on themselves than on others and often can more easily give and receive forgiveness than forgive themselves. But as individuals are able to accept their own humanity and forgive their errors and learn from them, they can apply that same understanding and compassion to others (Enright & Human Development Study Group, 1996).

FORGIVENESS IN SITUATIONS OF ILLNESS

Related to forgiveness for people with serious illness such as cancer, there has been little published work. One study of note was a phenomenologic study of the lived experiences of cancer patients who participated in a group forgiveness therapy (Phillips & Osborne, 1989). The findings support the value of forgiveness work through the patients' "journey of forgiveness" from their initial diagnosis; confrontation with the disease; struggle with guilt, blame, anger, and finding personal meaning; to the development of new insights and understanding.

There is, unfortunately, scant research on forgiveness to guide clinical application in serious illness populations; however, there is substantive work, particularly theoretical, in philosophy, theology, and psychology that, taken together, can guide its application to the many situations in oncology where forgiveness is an important issue for our patients.

CLINICAL IMPLICATIONS

Some of our patients may struggle with issues related to forgiveness; for example, some patients direct anger at themselves, others, the disease, or God, and for some, self-blame or other-blame create distress. Similarly, family members may be coping with forgiveness issues of their own. Viewing forgiveness from the perspective of "ceasing to feel angry or resentful towards" someone or something (Thompson, 1996, p. 343), we can apply forgiveness interventions within the oncology setting when appropriate and useful for our patients.

ASSESSING THE NEED FOR FORGIVENESS

How do we determine whether forgiveness is an issue for our patients? Seamands (1981) suggests three tests to help identify the need for forgiveness: (1) the resentment test (if the patient is resentful, hurt, or angry), (2) the responsibility test (if the patient is blaming someone or something for the illness), and (3) the reminder and reaction test (if the patient is reacting negatively to a current situation because of past unresolved issues). We should assess the patient's regrets, resentments, and reactions; identify areas that are causing distress; assist patients to come to terms with the issues; and support their resolution. Some patient examples are illustrative:

 I feel so badly that I am sick. I'm a young man who should be protecting and providing for his family. Instead I'm bringing them terrible pain and worry. I ask for my wife's forgiveness on a daily basis.

My body let me down. I exercise, eat well, take good care of myself and then I get cancer. I feel betrayed and angry.

I am dealing with a lot of personal regrets. I feel so guilty. I blame myself for my disease. I am having a hard time accepting this.

It's funny. Well, it might be funny if it weren't so painful. I don't even think about my cancer now. The thing that is always on my mind is the abuse that I had to endure from my father when I was a child. I get so enraged at him now. I can't understand it—that was so many years ago.

I am so angry at God. Why did He do this to me? Why did He give me of all people this terrible illness? I am a good person. I go to church every Sunday. I treat others with respect. I've never harmed anyone. What about all those people who rob, murder, rape? Why don't they have cancer?

My kids are so angry at me for being sick. They say you don't do things for us 'like you're supposed to, like other mothers . . . We can't go on vacations. We can't spend money. We can't go out because we have to help you around the house. And, all you do is lay around and complain about how sick you are.' They have no idea how they hurt me so deeply.

THE PROCESS OF FORGIVING

As oncology clinicians, we need to be aware of the situations in which forgiveness is important for patients and to help them understand the psychological process of forgiving. First and most important, forgiveness requires self-awareness (Meek & McMinn, 1997) of the anger and hurt and then experiencing the associated emotional pain (Enright, 1996). There is some evidence that patients who acknowledge their emotional pain and assume responsibility for their negative feelings are better able to release those feelings through forgiveness (Phillips & Osborne, 1989). Thus, we need to support patients with the necessary grief work surrounding illness-related losses, regrets, resentments, and anger, but caution patients not to rush to forgive too quickly. They must first experience and work through these associated emotions. Support patients as they identify, understand, and release negative feelings and attitudes.

ATTRIBUTION RETRAINING

Once the feelings have been experienced, patients can begin to see the actual issues more clearly. Because individuals' ability to forgive may be influenced by their attributions or personal judgments, various cognitive techniques such as reframing and attribution retraining, that is, changing one's thinking about the cause of events, may be helpful to facilitate the process of forgiveness (Al-Mabuk et al., 1998). This may involve correcting patients' faulty assumptions about disease causation and personal responsibility, about the intentions and motivations of others, or challenging damaging self-attributions of failure and inadequacy. Once negative attributions are identified and restructured with more constructive, positive explanations, individuals often are able to alter the perceptions that caused them distress and allow for new solutions and behaviors (Lawson, 1993) and for the hurtful event to be understood in a new perspective (Al-Mabuk et al., 1998).

CONFLICT RESOLUTION

Concerning relationships with others, Droll (1984) notes that forgiveness is essentially a conflict-resolution process. As Mermann (1992) has observed, patients with cancer have a gift denied many others—some time to prepare for the eventual end of life. This time can be used to bring old interpersonal conflicts to a close and to give and seek forgiveness from others. Illness should be a time for reconciliation and reckoning (Rinpoche, 1994). Encourage patients to come to terms with the conflicted relationships that are causing them distress. Guide patients to identify misunderstandings that are important to resolve for themselves and for their loved ones. Assist patients to come to a compassionate understanding of others' needs and frailties that may have contributed to these relationship conflicts, as well as the role they may have played in the conflict. Some patients may need assistance to recognize the importance of receiving forgiveness from others for hurts that they may have caused or to which they contributed (Enright & Human Development Study Group, 1996).

THE RECIPROCAL NATURE OF FORGIVENESS

Help patients understand the reciprocal nature of self-forgiveness and forgiveness of others. The greater the personal understanding and acceptance of one's own shortcomings, the greater the empathy with others, and the less harsh the judgments of self and others will be (Al-Mabuk et al., 1998; McCullough et al., 1997). Finally, assist patients to sort out what negativity ought to be directed at the disease and what is rightly directed at others. Patients may misplace anger directed at the cancer onto others (Phillips & Osborne, 1989), particularly those closest to and most needed by the patient. Assist patients in its appropriate resolution.

ANTICIPATING CONFLICTS

Relevant to the disease, providing information and correcting misunderstandings about cancer, its causes, its treatment, and prognosis are important strategies. Patients and family members need to develop a realistic understanding of the illness situation, their own reactions, and the reactions of others. For example, before beginning treatment, a family meeting may help to explain the side effects of treatment (eg, fatigue, nausea) so that the patient and family have clear, realistic expectations; the impact of the patient's disease and treatment on the family is acknowledged; and the patient can be supported with household or job responsibilities. Throughout treatment, keep the lines of communication open to correct misinformation, and offer support to patients and family members as they work through various illness-related issues and conflicts to come to terms with the disease and its effects. Guide the patient and family to identify and grieve the losses and changes necessitated by the disease, to set reasonable goals, and to problem solve workable solutions, particularly during times of transition in the course of the disease and shifts in treatment goals.

CORRECTING MISCONCEPTIONS

Related to self-forgiveness, identify issues of self-blame, and correct patients' misperceptions of disease causation and personal responsibility. Support patients to learn from their mistakes and to be gentle in their self-judgments. Patients' self-disclosure through the telling of their story may be important for self-forgiveness and resolution of self-blame. This sharing can be healing because a process of reintegration may take place, that is reintegrating parts of themselves that were split off and hidden because they were painful, shameful, and unacceptable (Ornish, 1998). The forgiveness goals are for patients to come to recognize their dignity and self-worth, to release blame and guilt, and to connect more affirmingly and meaningfully with others.

SUPPORTING THE WORK OF FORGIVENESS

It is imperative that we identify the spiritual needs of our patients and offer ongoing support to connect to personally meaningful religious or spiritual beliefs, cultural practices, or philosophical teachings that support forgiveness. Relaxation, meditation, prayer, positive affirmations, and journal writing are among the other strategies that may be helpful for patients to release anger and hurt directed at themselves, their illness, or others to facilitate the forgiveness process. Through the process of forgiveness of self and others, a new "world view" may be found, letting go of hurts, regrets, and resentments; accepting a common humanity; and experiencing inner peace, lowered distress, and improved quality of life (Phillips & Osborne, 1989).

OUR CONTRIBUTIONS TO SUPPORT FORGIVENESS

By valuing our patients, respecting their individuality, and acknowledging their needs without judgment, we as professional caregivers can provide relationships of support, trust, and care for our patients. We can offer personal acceptance through our actions and create a climate for the client and family that facilitates letting go of resentment, anger, hurt, and self-blame, which is essential to the forgiveness process (Hope, 1987; Benson, 1992).

THE VIOLATION OF ILLNESS

The "violation of illness" that the cancer may represent for some patients can be a powerful reawakening of earlier traumas or violations of personal integrity that have not been completely grieved or processed and now need to be re-experienced and forgiven. If issues of forgiveness are related to longstanding and significant personal or interpersonal conflicts or issues of blame, abuse, and violation, refer to psychological, psychiatric, or family counseling. If issues are related to a crisis of spiritual beliefs and religious conflicts, refer to religious or spiritual counseling.

In summary, forgiveness work is important as a supportive technique in oncology. It is important to acknowledge the personal hurt and resentment associated with cancer and the related interpersonal conflicts and difficulties and offer guidance for patients to take responsibility to do whatever is personally meaningful to cope positively with the disease without being consumed with anger, self-pity, blame, and self-recriminations.

CLINICAL STRATEGIES

1. Understand the patient's needs and objectives for forgiveness work. Patients must take personal responsibility and make choices about matters of forgiveness.
2. Guide patients to work through illness-related forgiveness issues.
3. When forgiveness issues involve past situations of severe trauma, for example abuse, rape, or incest, or are creating significant distress, refer to psychiatric, psychological, or family counseling.
4. When issues are related to a crisis of faith and religious beliefs, refer to spiritual or religious counseling.
5. Assist patients to identify and emotionally release anger, pain, and resentment over illness-related losses and changes.
6. Assist patients to understand the reactivation and contribution of past events to current distress.
7. Guide patients to understand their reactions to the disease and develop empathy to their own and others' shortcomings. Help them let go of the need for anger or blame.
8. Provide education and information to clarify misconceptions, misinformation, and inaccurate assumptions.
9. Forgiveness is a process that ultimately can lead people to convert their suffering into a personally meaningful and healing event (Ferch, 1998).
10. Because forgiveness is essentially a conflict resolution process (Droll, 1984), assist patients to come to terms with personal and interpersonal issues that are causing distress.
11. Make patients aware that issues of forgiveness may be important to identify and discuss, particularly if anger, hurt, and resentment are causing distress.

CASE STUDY

Mary, a 45-year-old patient with advanced lung cancer, was struggling with a very grim prognosis. Bob, her estranged husband of several years moved back into her home to help care for her and their two children. Their relationship had been quite conflicted over the years with many issues never discussed, let alone resolved. Mary and Bob came to see the oncology counselor for one visit to discuss the needs of the children before the patient's rapid decline and death. During this visit, after discussing the needs of their sons, the patient turned to Bob and told him that she was sorry for her contribution to their problems of the past. She asked his forgiveness and explained how deeply she appreciated his love, care, and support during this terrible illness. Bob was stunned. He was full of gratitude and admiration for her and offered his own apologies for his past behaviors and poor judgment. As a direct result of the forgiveness that Bob received, he was able to grieve her death effectively and was released from overwhelming guilt and ambivalence that could have impeded such important grief work.

REFERENCES

Al-Mabuk, R. H., Dedrick, C. V. L., & Vanderah, K. M. (1998). Attribution retraining in forgiveness therapy. *Journal of Family Psychotherapy, 9*(1), 11–30.

Augsburger, D. (1981). *Caring enough to forgive.* Ventura, CA: Regal Books.

Benson, C. (1992). Forgiveness and the psychotherapeutic process. *Journal of Psychology and Christianity, 11*(1), 76–81.

Bloch, D. (1992). *I am with you always: A treasury of inspirational quotations, poems, and prayers.* New York: Bantam Books.

Davenport, D. S. (1991). The functions of anger and forgiveness: Guidelines for psychotherapy with victims. Special Issue: Psychotherapy with victims. *Psychotherapy, 28*(1), 140–144.

Droll, D. M. (1984). *Forgiveness: Theory and research.* Unpublished doctoral dissertation, University of Nevada, Reno.

Enright, R. D., & Human Development Study Group, USA. (1996). Counseling within the forgiveness triad: On forgiving, receiving, forgiveness, and self-forgiveness. *Counseling and Values, 40*(2), 107–126.

Farmer, S. (1989). *Adult children and abusive parents.* Los Angeles: Lowell House.

Ferch, S. R. (1998). Intentional forgiving as a counseling intervention. *Journal of Counseling and Development, 76,* 261–270.

Fitzgibbons, R. P. (1986). The cognitive and emotive uses of forgiveness in the treatment of anger. *Psychotherapy, 23*(4), 629–633.

Freedman, S. R., & Enright, R. D. (1996). Forgiveness as an intervention with incest survivors. *Journal of Consulting and Clinical Psychology, 64,* 983–992.

Haber, J. G. (1991). *Forgiveness.* Savage, MD: Rowman and Littlefield.

Hebl, J. H., & Enright, R. D. (1993). Forgiveness as a psychotherapeutic goal with elderly females. *Psychotherapy, 30,* 658–667.

Holmgren, M. (1993). Forgiveness and the intrinsic value of persons. *American Philosophical Quarterly, 30,* 341–352.

Hope, D. (1987). The healing paradox of forgiveness. *Psychotherapy, 24,* 240–244.

Johnson, D. R., Feldman, S. C., Lubin, H., & Southwick, S. M. (1995). The therapeutic use of ritual and ceremony in the treatment of post-traumatic stress disorder. *Journal of Traumatic Stress, 8*(2).

Kaplan, B. H. (1992). Social health and the forgiving heart: The type B story. *Journal of Behavioral Medicine, 15,* 3–14.

Lawson, D. (1992). The family regulator of change reframe. In T. S. Nelson & T. S. Trepper (Eds.), *101 interventions in family therapy.* New York: The Haworth Press.

McCullough, M. E., Worthington, E. L., Jr., & Rachal, K. C. (1997). Interpersonal forgiving in close relationships. *Journal of Personality and Social Psychology, 73*(2), 321–336.

Meek, K. R., & McMinn, M. R. (1997). Forgiveness: More than a therapeutic technique. *Journal of Psychology and Christianity, 16*(1), 51–61.

Mermann, A. C. (1992). Spiritual aspects of death and dying. *Yale Journal of Biology & Medicine, 65*(2), 137–142.

Ornish, D. (1998). *Love and survival.* New York: Harper Perennial.

Phillips, L. J., & Osborne, J. W. (1989). Cancer patients' experiences of forgiveness therapy. *Canadian Journal of Counseling, 23*(3), 236–251.

Pingleton, J. P. (1997). Why we don't forgive: A biblical and object relations theoretical model for understanding failure in the forgiveness process. *Journal of Psychology and Theology, 25*(4), 403–413.

Rilke, R. M. (1930). *Notebooks of Malta.* London: Hogarth Press.

Ritzman, T. A. (1987). Forgiveness—its role in therapy. *Medical Hypnoanalysis Journal, 2,* 4–13.

Seamands, D. A. (1981). *Healing for damaged emotions.* Wheaton, IL: Victor Books.

Stoop, D. (1991). Forgiving our parents: Forgiving ourselves. Ann Arbor, MI: Vine.

Thompson, D. (Ed.) (1996). *The Oxford dictionary of current English.* New York: Oxford University Press.

Worthington, E. L., Jr., & DiBlasio, F. A. (1990). Promoting mutual forgiveness within the fractured relationship. *Psychotherapy, 27,* 219–223.

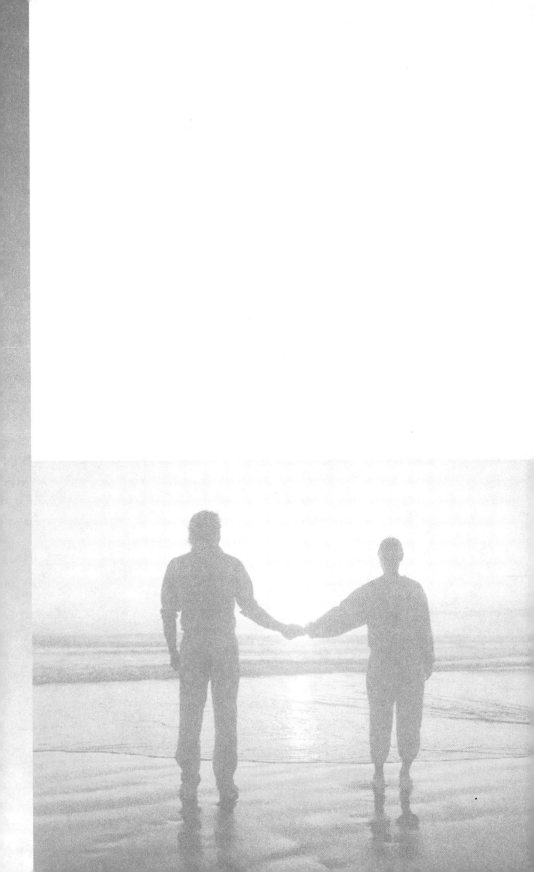

CHAPTER 9

Overview of Assessment and Management Strategies

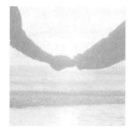

The purpose of this final chapter is to present a compilation of general psychosocial assessment and management guidelines for the treatment of depression and anxiety that are concise, useful, and practical for oncology clinicians. It also provides some examples of relaxation and meditation practices

ASSESSMENT OF DEPRESSIVE SYMPTOMATOLOGY

In general, most patients with cancer cope remarkably well with their illness and treatments. The most common psychological reactions are depression and anxiety (Massie & Holland, 1990). Sadness and grief are expected normal reactions to cancer. However, it is important for clinicians to distinguish sadness from depressive disorders. Symptoms of depression may cover a wide spectrum of responses ranging from "being blue" to major depressive disorders. If the symptoms become intense, protracted, and interfere with daily functioning, patients should be evaluated for major depression. Patients must be carefully and comprehensively evaluated, including psychological assessment of symptoms, physical evaluation, and review of lab data, medication and treatment effects, and past medical and psychiatric history (PDQ statement on depression, 1998). Some general assessment questions that may be useful to include in patients' psychosocial assessment follow:

- How do you view your illness?
- What is the meaning of your illness in your life and the lives of your significant others?
- How has cancer changed your life—positively or negatively?
- Describe your emotional reactions to your illness.
- Are these similar to or different from your usual style of reacting to situations?
- Do you cry? If yes, how often? Is this your usual response when faced with upsetting events? Do you feel better or worse after you cry?
- What other stressors are occurring in your life?
- What emotional support do you rely on? Is it sufficient?
- Are your spiritual or religious beliefs or practices an important source of comfort for you?
- Have you ever had episodes of depression? If so, describe the presentation, frequency, treatment, and resolution of the depressive episodes.

- How well do you think you are coping with your cancer?
- Have you felt sad, down, or had the "blues"?
- If yes, how long have you felt sad?
- How intense are these feelings? Do they interfere with your ability to function?
- If so, how? For example, have you had sleep, appetite, memory, concentration, or interpersonal problems?
- Do you feel hopeful?
- Do you feel worthwhile?
- Do you feel guilty?
- Have you felt pleasure or interest in doing things that are usually enjoyable for you?
- Do you ever feel so sad that you have thought about harming yourself?
- Do you have thoughts of suicide?
- If yes, have you thought about how you would actually harm yourself?
- Do you intend to harm yourself?
- Do you have a plan in mind?
- If so, could you tell me about it?
- Have you ever tried to harm yourself?

If patients have suicidal ideation, intent, and plan, they should immediately be referred (with safety precautions in place) to a psychiatrist or other mental health professional for evaluation and treatment. Following are other indications for psychiatric referral: The oncologist is not comfortable treating the patient's depression; the depressive symptoms are resistant to pharmacologic interventions after 4 to 6 weeks of treatment; the depressive symptoms are worsening rather than improving; the side effects of the medication prohibit therapeutic dosing of the antidepressant; or the symptoms are interfering with medical treatment (PDQ statement on depression, 1998).

DEVELOPING A TREATMENT PLAN

Based on the assessment data, a treatment plan should be collaboratively developed with the patient by determining concerns, issues, and needs in order of priority; including strategies the patient views as useful; and goals for treatment. Ascertain if the patient would like to speak with someone about emotional concerns, spiritual or existential issues, or family concerns. Ask patients what types of support would be most beneficial to them (eg, talking to their nurse or doctor, one-on-one psychological counseling, spiritual support, support groups, pastoral counseling, stress management training, educational groups, family counseling, mind–body training).

RISK FACTORS FOR DEPRESSION

Risk factors for depression in people with cancer include history of depression, poorly controlled pain, family history of depression or suicide, previous suicide attempts, history of alcoholism or drug abuse, advanced stage of cancer, increased physical impairment or discomfort, pancreatic cancer, concurrent illnesses that produce depressive symptoms, and treatment with certain chemotherapeutic agents (eg, vincristine, vinblastine, procarbazine, l-asparaginase, interferon, and amphotericin-b, and corticosteroids) and other medications (eg, tamoxifen, cimetidine, diazepam, and levodopa) (Massie, 1990).

MAJOR DEPRESSIVE EPISODE

If five or more of the following symptoms of depression are present during the same 2-week period and represent a change from previous functioning, with at least one of the symptoms being either depressed mood or loss of interest and pleasure, then a diagnosis of a major depressive episode can be made. These symptoms include depressed mood for most of the day and on most days as indicated either by patient report or by others (eg, patient is often tearful); diminished pleasure or interest in most activities; significant change in appetite and sleep patterns and fatigue (not explained by disease or treatment), psychomotor agitation, or slowing; feelings of worthlessness or excessive, inappropriate guilt; poor concentration; and recurrent thoughts of death (not just fear of dying) or suicide (American Psychiatric Association, 1994).

MANAGEMENT ISSUES

For patients with depressive symptoms related to their illness, the following suggestions may be helpful: using brief supportive counseling to help patients normalize their feelings, mobilizing support, minimizing stressors, using adaptive coping skills that have worked well in the past, and providing an opportunity for discussion of thoughts and feelings either through individual counseling or support groups.

TREATMENT OF MAJOR DEPRESSION

The recommended treatment of major depression is a combination of pharmacotherapy and psychotherapy. A patient's prior response to treatment is a useful predictor of the anticipated current response, so ascertain if patients have been treated successfully in the past for depression. Most common, the serotonin-specific reuptake inhibitors (SSRIs) are used to treat depression in patients with cancer, because they have few anticholenergic or cardiovascular side effects. Start with lower doses than used in healthy individuals with depression, and gradually increase the dose as needed for optimal therapeutic response. These antidepressants usually take approximately 4 weeks to have a therapeutic effect. Thus, the therapeutic effectiveness should not be evaluated until the patient has taken the SSRIs as prescribed for at least 4 to 6 weeks (Cutler & Marcus, 1999). The SSRIs include the following:

- Celexa (citalopram hydrobromide); dosage: 10 mg/d to start, then 20 to 40 mg/d
- Zoloft (sertraline); dosage: 25 mg/d to start, then 50 to 200 mg/d
- Paxil (paroxetine); dosage: 10 mg/d to start, then 20 to 50 mg/d
- Prozac (fluoxetine); dosage: 10 mg/d to start, then 20 to 80 mg/d

Counseling is usually managed with some combination of crisis intervention, medical crisis counseling, brief supportive therapy, cognitive and behavioral techniques, insight-oriented therapy, couple and family counseling, and self-help groups. These therapies explore methods of enhancing coping skills, lowering distress, supporting grief work, teaching problem-solving skills and stress management techniques, mobilizing support, reshaping negative or self-defeating thoughts, and developing a close bond with a knowledgeable empathic health professional (Massie, 1990; Massie & Holland, 1990; PDQ statement on depression, 1998).

ASSESSMENT OF ANXIETY

Anxiety often occurs in individuals with cancer and is a normal aspect of adapting to the disease. Anxiety is a normal reaction to that which is threatening to an individual's physical well-being, lifestyle, values, or loved ones. In most cases, the reactions are time limited and serve as a defense and warning for patients to prepare for a stressful life event. Anxiety at mild or moderate levels is normal in response to significant life stressors. Initial management includes providing adequate information and support to the patient. However, excessive or prolonged anxiety that interferes with normal functioning must be evaluated and treated. To evaluate anxiety, ask patients general questions about the presence, frequency, and intensity of anxiety and how much it interferes with daily living.

- How is the patient's anxiety manifested psychologically (eg, worry, tension, nervousness) and physically (eg, palpitations, sweating, difficulty breathing)?
- Does the patient have anxiety attacks, panic attacks? If so, how often, how intense, how disruptive, and what helps to relieve these attacks?
- Is there any discernible pattern to these attacks?
- Has the patient experienced anxiety disturbances in the past? If so, have the patient describe type, circumstances, and treatment.

Evaluate any medical reasons for heightened anxiety in patients, and refer to mental health professionals when anxiety has been intense, disruptive, long-standing, or has not responded to treatment (Massie, 1990; PDQ statements on depression and anxiety, 1998).

RISK FACTORS

The risk factors for anxiety disturbances include history of anxiety disorders, uncontrolled pain, functional limitations, lack of social support, advanced illness, and certain medical conditions (eg, abnormal metabolic states, hormone-secreting tumors), or medications (eg, corticosteroids, neuroleptics used as antiemetics, bronchodilators) (Massie, 1990).

MANAGEMENT ISSUES

Management includes a comprehensive assessment, physical and psychological evaluation, and accurate diagnosis. When anxiety is situational, that is caused by pain, underlying medical condition, or medication, then prompt treatment of the cause is necessary. General techniques to treat anxiety include a combination of pharmacotherapy (depending on severity of symptoms) and counseling. The counseling strategies generally used include cognitive-behavioral techniques, medical crisis counseling, brief supportive counseling, couple and family therapy, self-help groups, and behavioral interventions, such as relaxation training, guided imagery, and meditation exercises (PDQ statement on anxiety, 1998).

The anxiolytic medications most commonly used are the benzodiazepines. The choice of a benzodiazepine depends on a number of factors, such as the duration of action best suited to the patient, the rapidity of onset needed, the route of administration available, and metabolic problems to be considered. Dosing schedule depends on the patient's tolerance and requires individual titration. The shorter-acting benzodiazepines are alprazolam (Xanax) and lorazepam (Ativan) and the longer-acting include diazepam (Valium) and clonazepam (Klonopin) (Massie, 1990; PDQ statement on anxiety).

GENERAL COUNSELING INTERVENTIONS

Some general counseling approaches that may be useful for clinicians include understanding the needs and fears that are driving the patient's behavior; appreciating the personal meaning of the illness in the patient's life; being aware of the emotional range and limits of the patient; guiding the patient to use personal strengths; validating and witnessing the patient's emotional pain; supporting the necessary grieving or positively reframing the illness event in response to the patient's needs; respecting individual beliefs, values, and personal coping styles;

recognizing the need for defensive coping and the purpose it serves during threatening times; and offering new insights and teaching new ways of coping to those who are receptive to such strategies.

We need to recognize that the clinician's ability to connect, to relate to patients, is the most important variable in the professional relationship. Whiston and Sexton (1993), in a review of studies analyzing the efficacy of counseling relationships and patient outcomes, have found that it was not the specific techniques alone that produced positive outcomes for patients, but rather the relationship that was vital for personal growth. Techniques are secondary in that they occur within the interpersonal context of a supportive and caring relationship.

SOME THOUGHTS ON COMPASSION

Compassion perhaps is the most important single therapeutic characteristic when caring for individuals with cancer. One way to cultivate compassion in ourselves is to recognize the interconnection of all human beings. When someone is suffering and you find yourself at a loss to know how to help, Rinpoche (1994) advises that you put yourself unflinchingly in his or her place. Imagine as vividly as possible what you would be going through if you were suffering the same pain. Ask yourself how you would feel. How would you want your nurses and doctors to treat you? What would you want most from them? As Rinpoche (1994, p. 197) notes, "When you exchange yourself for others in this way, you are directly transferring your cherishing from its usual object, yourself, to other beings. So, exchanging yourself for others is a very powerful way of releasing the heart of your compassion."

Another moving technique for arousing compassion is to imagine one of your dearest friends, mother, father, husband, wife, child, or partner in the same kind of painful situation, and quite naturally your heart will open and compassion will awaken in you. You will find that your help is inspired more naturally and that you can direct it to patients more easily. Caring for the sick and dying makes us poignantly aware not only of their mortality, but also of our own. When we finally recognize this, we start to have an impassioned sense of the fragility and preciousness of each moment and each being, and from this can grow a deep, clear, limitless compassion for all human beings, as well as the determination to do all that is possible to care for them (Rinpoche, 1994).

HUMILITY

Finally, as clinicians, we ought to be humble to appreciate that our patients have tremendous inner resources. They know where they need to go and how best to get there. While they may need our guidance, support, and assistance during difficult times, we must rely on them to show us the direction and course that are best for them.

> Each of us must take responsibility for unraveling the mystery of our own lives, leaving to others the final responsibility for unraveling theirs . . . We can share our search with each other, we can help each other, but we cannot presume to have ultimate knowledge of each other's purposes and right directions. (Brown, 1983, p. 112).

REFERENCES

American Psychiatric Association. (1994). *Diagnostic and statistical manual of mental disorders* (4th ed.). Washington, D.C.: Author.

Brown, M. (1983). *The unfolding self.* Los Angeles: Psychosynthesis Press.

Cutler, J. L., & Marcus, E. R. (1999). *Psychiatry.* Philadelphia: W.B. Saunders.

Massie, M. J. (1990). Anxiety, panic, and phobias. In J. C. Holland & J. H. Rowland (Eds.), *Handbook of psychooncology* (pp. 300–309). New York: Oxford University Press.

Massie, M. J. (1990). Depression. In J. C. Holland & J. H. Rowland (Eds.), *Handbook of psychooncology* (pp. 283–290). New York: Oxford University Press.

Massie, M. J., & Holland, J. C. (1990). Overview of normal reactions and prevalence of psychiatric disorders. In J. C. Holland & J. H. Rowland (Eds.), *Handbook of psychooncology* (pp. 273–282). New York: Oxford University Press.

PDQ statements on depression and anxiety. (1998). [On-line cancer information]. Bethesda, MD: International Cancer Information Center, National Cancer Institute.

Rinpoche, S. (1994). *The Tibetan book of living and dying* (pp. 73–74). San Francisco: Harper.

Whiston, S. C., & Sexton, T. L. ((1993). An overview of psychotherapy outcome research. *Implications for practice, 24*(1), 43–51.

General Interventions, According to Life Stage to Be Used as a Guide for Clinicians

Intervention to Aid Coping With Cancer-Related Emotional Distress

Life Stage	Altered Personal Relationships	Issues of Dependence and Independence
Young adults (ages 19–30)	• Encourage hospital and home family visits. • Encourage role functions that can be maintained (decision making, child care activities). • Offer guidance and support as to what information about illness should be given to children, parents, friends, and colleagues. • Assess patient's relationship with key person sharing illness • Encourage counseling and attendance at young adult support groups regarding attitudes, beliefs, and feelings about cancer. • Encourage planning for family security (wills, substitute caregivers).	• Perform early assessment of rehabilitative potential to prevent the fixation of maladaptive responses (overdependence, poor motivation, unrealistic expectations or efforts).

Continued

Disruption of Achievement	Impairment of Health, Body Image, and Sexuality	Existential Issues
• Offer help in redefining life goals after illness. • Encourage clarification of job security (sick leave entitlement, disability). • Encourage review and refinancing of liabilities and obligations.	• Explore meaning of illness to individual's sense of self-worth and future. • Adapt sex counseling therapies to special problems and needs.	• Offer pastoral counseling.

Intervention to Aid Coping With Cancer-Related Emotional Distress—cont'd

Life Stage	Altered Personal Relationships	Issues of Dependence and Independence
Mature adults (ages 31–45)	• Maintain normal patterns of home life and activities of daily living (ADL). • Foster visits by family, friends, and peers; counsel about interpersonal relationships. • Provide groups of patients or significant others to deal with shared feelings about illness and goals and with negative information or attitudes about cancer. • Aid access to financial planning for illness and decreased income. • Refer patient to social services department for home care as necessary. • Communicate with children about parent's illness. Monitor their responses and facilitate opportunities to talk with parent.	• Encourage maximal self-care. • Promote concrete rehabilitation goals involving the patient's self-care, striving for as normal as possible living and working conditions. • Encourage patient to feel partnership in care with physician. • Facilitate counseling by "veteran patient."
Mature adults (ages 46–65)	• Provide referral for social services consultation regarding family and patient welfare. • Evaluate social support systems and facilitate alternative resources where lacking. • Consider joint or personal therapy to deal with conflicts about disease and death.	• Institute rehabilitative measures necessary to achieve maximal independence. • Provide assistance with ADL as needed. • Encourage patient to tolerate dependence on others when required. • Explore available financial resources and alternatives for nursing care if needed.

Disruption of Achievement	Impairment of Health, Body Image, and Sexuality	Existential Issues
• Facilitate return to home, school, or job as quickly as possible with rehabilitation and retraining as necessary. • Provide referral for counseling to help patient adjust to goal limitations.	• Support normal appearance and function (wigs, prostheses, clothes, make-up). • Make referral for sex counseling for patient or couple. • Refer couple for fertility/adoption advice if desired. • Use "veteran patient" models to offer reassurance through physical examinations to combat anxiety about recurrent disease.	• Facilitate patient's search for meaning of past and remaining life, death, and afterlife.
• Offer counseling that focuses on grief associated with loss of hoped-for lifestyle and goals. • Encourage realistic financial planning.	• Give special attention to well-fitted prostheses. • Offer counseling for practical management of altered physical appearance and body functions. • Promote good and regular personal hygiene. • Refer patient for psychiatric evaluation of severe depressive symptoms. • Explain side effects of treatment. • Offer reassurance about sexual identity despite distressing physical changes	• Encourage self-esteem-building life review. • Reinforce adaptive coping mechanisms and behaviors. • Expect patient to explore philosophical and religious meaning of life and death.

Continued

Intervention to Aid Coping With
Cancer-Related Emotional Distress—cont'd

Life Stage	Altered Personal Relationships	Issues of Dependence and Independence
Older adults (age 66 and older)	• Maintain, reestablish, or develop social support networks (religious, social, familial). • Stress need for orientation to new environments and treatments. • Stress continuity of care by trusted and familiar staff. • Support shared activities and affectional ties with family and friends.	• Strive for level of care that does not exceed patient's need. • Explore home or alternative care options (home visits, Meals on Wheels, nursing home, hospice). • Discuss feelings about dependence and helplessness.

(Adapted with permission from Houldin, A. D., & Lowery, B. J. [1992]. Emotional distress in breast cancer patients. *Med-Surg Nursing Quarterly,* 1[2], 6–13).

Disruption of Achievement	Impairment of Health, Body Image, and Sexuality	Existential Issues
• Expect counseling to focus on grief associated with loss of hoped-for-lifestyle and goals. • Encourage realistic financial planning (best use of available financial assets). • Tap community financial aid resources (Medicare, American Cancer Society). • Encourage meaningful hobbies and recreation.	• Plan daily routine with help as needed (bathing and so forth). • Obtain aids for sensory losses (if needed). • Aid time-and-place orientation (large clocks calendars, night-lights). • Encourage consistent caregivers and family support for sense of security. • Provide close monitoring for complications of illness and treatment.	• Allow discussion and plans about death, funeral, and burial, if desired. • Arrange visit with clergyman or chaplain. • Foster positive review of past life and achievements. • Offer supportive understanding of personal and physical losses.

Relaxation and Meditation Practices

BREATHING EXERCISE TO LET GO OF TENSION

1. Sit comfortably in a chair with your feet on the floor.
2. Breathe in deeply into your abdomen and say to yourself, "Breathe in relaxation." Pause before you exhale.
3. Breathe out from your abdomen and say to yourself, "Breathe out tension." Pause before you exhale.
4. Use each inhalation as a moment to become aware of any tension in your body.
5. Use each exhalation as an opportunity to let go of tension.
6. You may find it helpful to use your imagination to picture or feel the relaxation entering and the tension leaving your body (Davis, Eshelman, & McKay, 1995).

QUICK VERSION OF PROGRESSIVE MUSCLE RELAXATION

1. Curl both fists, tightening biceps and forearms. Relax.
2. Wrinkle up forehead. At the same time, press your head as far back as possible, roll it clockwise in a complete circle, and reverse. Now, wrinkle up the muscles of your face like a walnut: frowning, eyes squinted, lips pursed, tongue pressing the roof of your mouth, and shoulders hunched. Relax.
3. Arch back as you take a deep breath into the chest. Hold. Relax. Take a deep breath, pressing out the stomach. Hold. Relax.

4. Pull feet and toes back toward the face, tightening shins. Hold. Relax. Curl toes, simultaneously tightening calves, thighs, and buttocks. Relax (Davis et al., 1995, pp. 37–38).

LETTING GO OF THOUGHTS

1. Sit in a comfortable position, and take several deep breaths.
2. Close your eyes and imagine yourself comfortably sitting at the bottom of a deep pool of water. When you have a thought, feeling, or perception, see it as a bubble and let it rise away from you and disappear. When it's gone, wait for the next one to appear and repeat the process. Don't think about the contents of the bubble. Just observe it. Sometimes the same bubble may come up many times, or several bubbles will seem to be related to each other, or the bubbles may be empty. That's okay. Don't allow yourself to be concerned with these thoughts. Just watch them pass in front of your mind's eye.
3. If you feel uncomfortable imagining being under water, imagine that you are sitting on the bank of a river, watching a leaf drift slowly downstream. Observe one thought, feeling, or perception as the leaf, and then let it drift out of sight. Return to gazing at the river, waiting for the next leaf to float by with a new thought (Davis et al., 1995, p. 53).

INTRODUCTION TO THE PRACTICE OF MEDITATION

The purpose of meditation as Rinpoche (1994) has noted can be condensed into three crucial points: Bring your mind home; release; and relax. To release means to release your mind from its prison of grasping, because you recognize that all pain, fear, and distress arise from the craving of the grasping mind. To relax means to be spacious and to relax the mind of its tensions and worries. Relax into your true nature, letting all thoughts and emotions naturally subside and dissolve. Quietly sitting, body still, speech silent, mind at peace, let emotions and thoughts, whatever rises, come and go without clinging to anything, content simply to be fully present to yourself in the moment. The goal is to achieve a pure state of total presence. Once we have found this stability in meditation, disturbances of every kind will have far less impact. Rinpoche (1994) also points out that we have become too preoccupied by the "technology of meditation." What we need to appreciate is that the most important feature of meditation is not the technique, but rather the spirit. The skillful, inspired, and creative way in which we practice. Sometimes people think that when they meditate, there should be no thoughts or emotions at all, and when they arise people feel annoyed, frustrated, and think they have failed. This is not the case.

There is a Tibetan saying:

> It's a tall order to ask for meat without bones, and tea without leaves. So long as you have a mind, there will be thoughts and emotions. Just as the ocean has waves, so the mind's own radiance is its thoughts and emotions. The ocean has waves, but the ocean is not particularly disturbed by them. The waves are the very nature of the ocean. Waves will rise and then recede back into the ocean. In the same manner, the thoughts and emotions rise from the mind and dissolve back into the mind. Whatever rises, do not see it as a particular problem. If you do not impulsively react, if you are patient, it will once again settle into its essential nature. Don't grasp at it, feed it, or indulge it; don't cling to it and don't try to solidify it. Neither follow thoughts nor invite them; be like the ocean looking at its own waves with detached awareness, no judgment; just experience them and they will pass (Rinpoche, 1994, pp. 73–74).

MEDITATION PRACTICES

The following meditation practices were adapted with permission from *Pocketful of Miracles* by Joan Borysenko, PhD, which was originally adapted from *The Tibetan Book of Living and Dying* by Sogyal Rinpoche.

SHAMATHA/VIPASSANA MEDITATION

The Tibetan Buddhist practice of shamatha/vipassana, which means the meditation of calm abiding and insight, is a basic meditation practice.

Sit in your seat with great dignity, back straight and eyes open. Look directly in front of you, eyes down slightly, without particular focus. Become aware of your breathing—how breath comes in and fills you and how breath moves out into space. Keep about 25% of your attention on breathing and the other 75% on the feeling of spaciousness. When thoughts arise, just let them go by.

MINDFULNESS

A man who had a near-death experience following a heart attack returned to his body, and the first thing he saw in his hospital room was a rose. He experienced seeing a rose as for the first time, realizing that he was intimately connected to that flower. Now, when he walks through the forest, he feels as though he is one with the trees. He has realized directly his participation in the web of life. The secret of happiness, he says, is twofold: to realize that all things are interconnected and to send love along those connections. This attitude leads directly into the experience of mindfulness—the curious, open-minded observation of life that characterizes children.

Keeping your eyes open, take a deep breath and let go, feeling your body and mind begin to relax. Shift your attention to belly breathing. Look around and select an object to contemplate. Keeping an awareness of your breathing, see the object with the eyes of a child, as if you were seeing it for the first time. See with wonder, delight, and absorption. This is mindfulness, or moment-by-moment, nonjudgmental awareness.

Several times each day, stop and take a letting-go breath. Enter the moment with all your senses, taking time to taste and smell, hear and see, feel and move. Feel your connectedness with all things. Begin with a moment of mindfulness right now.

MINDFULNESS EXERCISES

We can extend the practice of mindful awareness and spaciousness beyond the period of sitting meditation into the rest of life. The Vietnamese Buddhist poet, peace-worker, and meditation teacher, Thich Nhat Hahn, has written a beautiful book called *The Miracle of Mindfulness*. With true simplicity and beauty, he reminds us that we can wake up in the ordinary activities of life by bringing our full attention to eating, washing the dishes, smelling the roses, walking.

Mindful eating: *Today, choose a piece of fruit and eat it mindfully. Be aware of its look, smell, and feel. Notice the way that your mouth fills with saliva in anticipation of its flavor. Be aware of each bite moving down your throat into your stomach.*

Mindful activity of your choice: *Choose one activity, like taking a walk, washing the dishes, or taking a shower, and commit to doing it as mindfully as possible.*

Mindfulness blessings (Brachot): A beautiful practice from Judaism is the recitation of blessings, called *Brachot*, which are prayers of gratitude. Judaism is similar to Greek Orthodoxy in being a tradition of gratitude to God for every kind of natural wonder—things that grow, stars that shine, rainbows, food we eat, even the natural functions of elimination that keep our bodies healthy. Brachot naturally brings us into mindfulness.

The bracha is a blessing of God for all that has been created. You can say an impromptu blessing whenever you notice something of wonder or beauty: Blessed art Thou, Creator of the Universe, who has given us the first star of evening, or the light of the moon, or the smile of babies. After each one, spend a minute or two in mindfulness and gratitude.

Mindful walking: *Place your attention lightly on the flow of your breathing. At the same time, notice how your body moves, how the weight shifts from one foot to the other. Perhaps you can coordinate your footsteps with your breathing, two or so steps to each in-breath and out-breath. The sensation of breathing and walking is like the anchor for your attention. When you feel focused in breathing and walking, open your senses to everything around you. The breath is like a bridge between you and everything you see, touch, smell, and sense. If your mind wanders, return to the sensation of breathing and walking.*

REFERENCES

Davis, M., Eshelman, E. R. & McKay, M. (1995). *The relaxation and stress reduction workbook* (p. 29). Oakland, CA: New Harbinger Publications.

Rinpoche, S. (1994). *The Tibetan book of living and dying.* San Francisco: Harper.

INDEX

A

adjustment
  control and, 61
  description of, 4
  hope and, 31
antidepressants, 129
anxiety
  assessment of, 130
  management of, 131
  risk factors, 130–131
assessments
  denial, 19–20
  depression, 126–127
  forgiveness, 115–116
  hope, 33
  need for control, 64–65
  uncertainty, 50–51
attribution
  in finding meaning, 95
  in forgiveness therapy, 112, 117
  principles of, 95
  in regaining control, 66
avoidance strategies, 104–105

B

benzodiazepines, 131

C

cancer
  meaning of. See meaning
  misconceptions regarding, 118–119
  psychological reactions and, 6
  psychoneuroimmunology research findings regarding, 5–6
  "violation" nature of, 119–120
caregiver. See also clinician; nurse; physician
  patient's needs during suffering, 83
  personal reflection by, 105–106
  role in forgiveness, 119
caring
  empathetic, 82
  sharing of suffering and, 82
case study examples
  control, 70–71

case study examples *(continued)*
   denial, 23–24
   forgiveness, 121
   hope, 39
   meaning, 106–107
   mind–body healing techniques, 10–11
   suffering, 88–89
   uncertainty, 55
causal thinking, 95
Celexa. See citalopram hydrobromide
chronic sorrow
   description of, 80–81
   interventions for, 85–86
citalopram hydrobromide, 129
clinician. See also caregiver; nurse; physician
   clinical reality presented by, 105
   denial by, 17–18, 22
   hope contributions by, 36–38
   patient's needs from, during suffering, 82–83
   personal reflection by, 105–106
   role in forgiveness, 119
   suffering of, 87
   vicarious control exercised by, 62–63, 66–67
cognitive adaptation model, 61
communication
   denial effects on, 22
   meaningful, 83–84
compassion, 84, 132
conflict
   anticipation of, 118
   forgiveness and, 117
   self-conflict, 77–78
   suffering and, 77–78
connections
   loss of, 85
   meaningful, 103–104
control
   adjustment and, 61
   assessing need for, 64–65
   burdens associated with, 62, 66, 68
   case study example of, 70–71
   causal attributions to regain, 66
   central, 61, 69
   clinical strategies for, 70
   consequence-related, 61, 69
   coping and, 60–61

cost–benefit analysis of, 68
distress levels and, 65
enhancing of, 69
hope and, 30
illusions of, 61–62, 68
loss of, 67, 70–71
for mitigating distress, 67–68
perceived, 60
reactions to loss of, 67
regaining, 8
relative need for, 63
relinquishing of, 64
self-determined individuals and, 64
self-efficacy and, 68–69
shifts in focus of, 69
variation in need for, 63–64
vicarious, 62–63, 66–67
coping
adaptive, 2–3
control and, 60–61
denial. See denial
facilitation of, 7
meaning and, 97, 101
questions, 7
for uncertainty, 46–47, 51–52
variations in, 7, 9
counseling
approaches for, 131–132
for depression, 129–130

D

denial
adaptive use, 18–19
approaches to, 16
assessment of, 19–20
case study example of, 23–24
clinical strategies for, 23
communication impediments secondary to, 22
confrontation of, 17, 20
dealing with, 20
definition of, 16–17, 19
expressing of, 20
by family members, 17
interpersonal nature of, 16–17, 19

denial *(continued)*
    isolating nature of, 22
    maladaptive use, 18, 20
    outcome research regarding, 18
    overview of, 16
    by patients, 17–19
    perception of, 21
    problems secondary to, 20
    as process, 18
    promoting of, 22
    for protecting family members, 21–22
    self-protective use of, 17
    by staff, 17–18, 22
    subjective interpretation of, 21
    treatment compliance effects, 16, 20
depression. See also major depressive episode
    assessment of, 126–127
    management of, 129
    risk factors, 128
    signs and symptoms of, 128
    treatment of, 127–130
despair
    adaptive nature of, 28–29
    false, 38
    hope and, 31
distress. See also upset
    clinical strategies for, 9–10
    expression of, 2
    family members, 8–9
    hope and, 34
    importance of, 4
    manifestation of, 3
    need for control and, 65
    normalizing of, 3, 8
    onset of, 4
    phases of, 3–4
    sense of purpose and, 96
    systemic effects of, 4–5
    uncertainty and, 46

E

emotional detachment, 4
emotions
    physiological effects, 5

types of, 6, 100–101
empathetic caring, 82
empathetic witnessing, 102

F

family members
    denial by, 17, 21–22
    distress of, 8–9
    hope from, 34, 36
    questions commonly asked by, 7
    strain on, 36
    suffering of, 86–87
    support for, 8–9
    uncertainty in, 49
feelings, 100–101
fluoxetine, 129
forgiveness
    assessing need for, 115–116
    attribution retraining and, 112, 117
    benefits of, 112
    case study example of, 121
    clinical strategies for, 120
    conflict-resolution nature of, 117
    definition of, 113–114
    in illness situations, 114–115
    importance of, 120
    individual differences in, 113
    integrated approach, 112
    need for, 115–116
    overview of, 115
    principles of, 112
    process of, 116
    reciprocal nature of, 118
    religious foundation of, 112–114
    research regarding, 112
    of self, 114, 118–119
    support for, 119
    therapeutic nature of, 113–114

G

grief, 31, 97, 103, 116

H

Herth Hope Scale, 33
hope
  adaptive nature of, 28–29
  assessment of, 33
  in cancer patients, 30–31
  case study example of, 39
  clinical strategies for, 38–39
  clinician's contributions, 36–37
  cognitive techniques for, 34
  control and, 30
  defining of, 29
  description of, 28
  despair and, 28–29, 31
  enhancing of, 32–36
  faith and, 30
  false, 38
  generalized, 29
  healing power of, 28
  information delivery and, 38
  loss of, 28
  maladaptive, 28, 31
  medical information truth telling and, 37–38
  mindfulness meditation technique, 35
  negative influences on, 37
  outcomes of, 29–30
  particularized, 29
  personal experience of, 29–30
  from the presence of others, 34
  process-related nature of, 31–32, 35
  realigning of, 32–33
  respect and, 37
  spiritual aspects of, 30
  subjective interpretation of, 29, 32
  sustaining of, 17–18, 30, 35–36
  symptom management and, 34–35
  truth and, conflicts between, 36
  unfulfilled, 36
humility, 133

I

illness. See cancer
illness-related uncertainty. See uncertainty, illness-related
information. See medical information

isolation
    denial and, 22
    loss of connection and, 85
    suffering and, 77, 85

M

major depressive episode. See also depression
    signs and symptoms of, 128
    treatment of, 129–130
meaning
    approaches to, 94
    attribution research findings, 95
    avoidance strategies, 104–105
    case study example of, 106–107
    clinical strategies for, 106
    coping styles and, 101
    discovery of, 101
    as dynamic process, 100–101
    empathetic witnessing and, 102
    grieving and, 103
    illness as a problem of, 98–99
    interventions, 101–102
    meaningful connections, 103–104
    mortality and, 97
    negative, 97–98
    nonexistent, 97–98
    overview of, 94
    personal, 94, 96
    questions for assessing, 98–99
    relative nature of, 96–97
    search for, 94–96
    sources of, 99
    story-telling for conveying, 102–103
    in suffering, 84–85
    unconditional, 104
    variations in, 98–100
meaningful communication, 83–84
meaningful connections, 103–104
medical information
    hope and, 38
    truth telling regarding, effect on hope, 37–38
meditation
    mindfulness, 35
    Tonglen, 85
mind–body study. See psychoneuroimmunology

mindfulness, 35
misconceptions, 118–119
mortality, 97

N

nurse. See also caregiver; clinician; physician
    denial as viewed by, 18
    patient's needs during suffering, 83
    suffering of, 87

P

paroxetine, 129
patients
    denial by, 17–19
    knowledge of psychoneuroimmunology by, 9
    perceptions of, 8
    questions commonly asked by, 7
Paxil. See paroxetine
perceived control, 60
personal meaning. See meaning
phases of response, to diagnosis, 3–4
physician. See also caregiver; clinician; nurse
    denial as viewed by, 17–18
    patient's needs from, during suffering, 83
    suffering of, 87
pity, 84
Prozac. See fluoxetine
psychological distress. See distress
psychoneuroimmunology
    cancer and, 5–6
    case study examples, 10–11
    contradictory nature of information regarding, 9, 11
    origins of, 5
    patient's understanding of, 9
    research findings, 5–6
psychosocial oncology care, 7

Q

questions
    for anxiety assessments, 130
    for assessing patient's view of illness, 98–99

commonly asked types of, 7
for depression assessments, 126–127

R

response phases, 3–4

S

self-conflict, 77–78
self-doubt, 2
self-efficacy, 68–69
self-forgiveness, 114, 118–119
serotonin-specific reuptake inhibitors, 129
sertraline, 129
social learning theory, 68
sorrow, chronic
    description of, 80–81
    interventions for, 85–86
spirituality
    hope and, 30
    identifying needs for, 119
    suffering and, 76
staff
    denial by, 17–18, 22
    suffering of, 87
stress
    neuroimmune changes and, 5–6
    physiological effects, 5–6
stressors
    control of. See control
    psychological nature of, 6
suffering
    case study example of, 88–89
    chronic sorrow and, 80–81, 85–86
    clinical strategies for, 88
    compassion for, 84, 132
    contributing factors, 80
    control of, 78–79
    definition of, 76
    of family members, 86–87
    individual interpretation of, 79, 81–82
    isolation secondary to, 77
    loss of connection secondary to, 85
    meaningful communication for, 83–84

suffering *(continued)*
  meaning in, 84–85
  nature of, 76–77
  patient's needs from caregiver during, 83
  personal context of, 81–82
  personal growth and, 78
  reasons for, 81
  relieving, 83
  scientific inquiry regarding, 76
  self-conflict and, 77–78
  sharing of, as method of caring, 82
  social nature of, 77
  sources of, 79–80
  spiritual dimension of, 76
  of staff, 87
  subjective nature of, 77, 79
  types of, 82
  value of, 78
  variations in, 81
suicidal ideation, 127
symptom management
  anxiety, 130–131
  depressive symptomatology. See depression
  hope and, 34–35

T

Tonglen, 85

U

uncertainty, illness-related
  appraisal of, 45–46
  assessment of, 50–51
  case study example of, 55
  categorization of, 47
  clinical strategies for, 54
  complex nature of, 49–50
  components of, 49–50
  coping strategies, 46–47, 51–52
  daily living, 47, 53
  as danger, 45–46, 50
  definition of, 44
  elements related to, 48–49
  etiologic, 47–48, 53
  exacerbations of, 51

exaggerated, 50
fear and, 52
living with, 52
management of, 53–54
medical, 47
as opportunity, 45–46, 50
outcomes research regarding, 44, 49
patterns of, 47–48
personal perception of, 45
positiveness of, 46–47
social support and, 49
strategies for reducing, 8, 52–53
symptom, 47, 53
vulnerability and, 45
unconditional meaning, 104
upset. See also distress
discovery of meaning, 101
normalizing of, 3, 8

V

vicarious control, 62–63, 66–67
vulnerability
suffering and, 87
uncertainty and, 45

Z

Zoloft. See sertraline